The Power Within: Discovering Your Motivation to Succeed

BY A.S.

TABLE OF CONTENTS

Book Title: The Power Within: Discovering Your Motivation to Succeed

DEDICATION

As I sit down to write this book, I can't help but feel overwhelmed by the love and gratitude I have for you. You are my rock, my partner, my best friend, and my soulmate. You have been there for me through thick and thin, through the ups and downs of life, and I cannot imagine where I would be without you. You are Truly my World.

I love you; A.S.

BOOK INTRODUCTION:

Life can be tough. It can challenge you in ways you never imagined, and it can be easy to lose motivation and give up. But what if you had the power within you to succeed, no matter what life throws your way? What if you could tap into a source of motivation that would keep you going through thick and thin?

This book is about discovering that power within you - the power of motivation. It's about unlocking your potential and tapping into your inner drive to succeed. Through the pages of this book, you'll discover the tools and techniques you need to overcome fear and doubt, find purpose and meaning, and cultivate positive habits that will sustain your motivation for the long haul.

Each chapter is designed to take you on a journey of self-discovery and personal growth. You'll explore the role of mindset in motivation, the power of passion and purpose, and the importance of community and environment. You'll learn how to overcome obstacles and build resilience, and how to cultivate gratitude and a positive outlook on life.

But most importantly, you'll learn how to tap into the power within you - the power of motivation - to achieve your goals and dreams. You'll discover that you have what it takes to succeed, no matter what life throws your way.

So if you're ready to discover the power within you and tap into your inner drive to succeed, then this book is for you. It's time to unleash your full potential and live the life you were meant to live.

Chapter 1

THE CALL TO ACTION

Dear Reader,

Have you ever felt stuck in life, like you're not living up to your full potential? Do you have dreams and goals that you've been putting off because you're afraid or unsure of how to achieve them? If so, then you're not alone. Many people struggle with motivation, and it can be tough to find the drive to take action and pursue your dreams.

But here's the thing - motivation is not something that just happens to you. It's something you have to create for yourself. It's a choice you make every day to take action, to push past your fears and doubts, and to pursue your goals with passion and purpose. Each day that you go on about your business is another chance to find the secret power that lives within you, When you open yourself to that power you will find the need to move and to change certain aspects of yourself, for you are human and

Human beings are not static by nature. we evolve depending on our conscious and unconscious will. Each new day that we inherit is a new opportunity to make the changes necessary in your life to find or to create a new you. once your recognize this fact you will feel a need to move, to change yourself from within, this is called the the call to action Lets briefly take the next few paragraphs and investigate this more in depth- the moment when you decide to take control of your life and create the motivation you need to succeed, is when the process of Healing and self redevelopment occur. No lets take a look at the power of choice and the importance of taking action, even when you're afraid or uncertain what comes to mind when you seek to change, is it fear of the unknown, or is it happiness that takes the fore. if it is the prior then feel comfort because you are not alone, everyone feels fear in the face of the unknown whether it is a fear of failure or a fear of letting yourself or your loved ones down it doesn't matter. Now if you happen to be within the small subset of humanity that is in the latter grouping, then you are a rare person, you have the soul of a warrior naturally. not saying that those in the first group are not warriors, it is just a matter of training and a matter of self discipline that creates the chasm which separates the two groups.

anyone can become a warrior given the tools to do so, however very few are born into this life already having the core values which create Warriors at the start. What exactly is the difference between these two groups, Time and Motivation, which leads us into your mindset.

We'll also explore the role of mindset in motivation. Your mindset - the way you think about yourself and your abilities - can have a huge impact on your motivation. If you believe that you're capable of achieving your goals, then you're more likely to take action and pursue them. But if you believe that you're not good enough or that you'll never succeed, then you're likely to hold yourself back. these two kinds of mindset are prevalent in most people, however if you take a second to consider your thoughts then you will realize that the only person truly holding you back is yourself.

The good news is that you can change your mindset. You can learn to believe in yourself and change the negative thoughts that plague you. Like no matter how hard you try, you just can't seem to break free from your own self-doubt and insecurities? If so, you're not alone. Many people struggle with negative thoughts and beliefs that hold them back from reaching their full potential.

But the good news is that you don't have to stay stuck in this pattern. You have the power to change your mindset and believe in yourself.

1: The Science of Positive Thinking

The research behind positive thinking and how it can benefit your mental and physical health. We'll delve into the neuroscience of the brain, and how positive thoughts can stimulate the release of feel-good hormones like dopamine and serotonin. We'll also look at the connection between positive thinking and stress reduction, and how a positive mindset can help you cope with challenging situations.The power of positive thinking is truly remarkable. It's amazing how our thoughts and beliefs can have such a profound impact on our mental and physical health. Positive thinking has been scientifically proven to stimulate the release of feel-good hormones like dopamine and serotonin in the brain, which can lead to improved mood, reduced stress, and increased overall well-being.

When we think positively, we're more likely to see opportunities instead of obstacles, and to approach challenges with a growth mindset. This can help us to cope better with stressful situations, and to bounce back more quickly from setbacks and disappointments. When we focus on the positive, we're better able to cultivate resilience, grit, and determination, which can help us to achieve our goals and dreams.

The neuroscience of the brain is truly fascinating. When we think positively, our brain produces more neural connections in the areas associated with happiness, optimism, and well-being. This means that the more we focus on the positive, the more our brain becomes wired to see the good in every situation, even in the face of adversity.

On the other hand, negative thinking can have a profound impact on our mental and physical health. When we focus on the negative, our brain produces more stress hormones like cortisol, which can lead to increased anxiety, depression, and other health issues. Negative thoughts can also lead to a fixed mindset, where we feel stuck and unable to overcome challenges or make positive changes in our lives.

So, the next time you find yourself caught in a cycle of negative thinking, remember the power of positive thinking. It's never too late to start shifting your mindset and focusing on the positive. By cultivating a more positive outlook, you can improve your mental and physical health, reduce stress, and increase your overall sense of well-being. So, take the time to focus on the good in your life, and watch as your mindset and your life begin to transform in amazing ways.

2: Identifying Negative Thoughts

Before you can change your mindset, it's important to first identify the negative thoughts and beliefs that are holding you back. Let's walk you through the process of identifying your negative self-talk, and provide you with practical strategies for challenging and reframing those thoughts. Identifying our negative thoughts and beliefs can be a daunting task, but it's an essential first step in changing our mindset and improving our overall well-being. Negative self-talk can be like a toxic voice inside our heads, telling us that we're not good enough, that we'll never succeed, or that we don't deserve happiness and success. This kind of self-talk can hold us back from reaching our full potential and achieving our dreams.

But the good news is that we have the power to change our negative self-talk and beliefs. The first step is to identify the negative thoughts and beliefs that are holding us back. This can be done by simply paying attention to our inner dialogue and the patterns of our thoughts. It can be helpful to keep a journal or log of our negative self-talk, so that we can see it more clearly and objectively.

Once we've identified our negative self-talk, it's important to challenge and reframe those thoughts. We can do this by asking ourselves questions like "Is this thought really true?" or "What evidence do I have to support this belief?" We can also try to reframe negative thoughts in a more positive light, by replacing them with affirmations or positive self-talk.

It's important to remember that changing our mindset takes time and practice. We may not be able to completely eliminate our negative self-talk overnight, but with consistent effort, we can begin to shift our thoughts and beliefs in a more positive direction.

By identifying and challenging our negative self-talk, we can begin to build a more positive mindset, and improve our overall well-being. We can start to see ourselves in a more positive light, and believe in our own potential for success and happiness. So, take the time to identify your negative self-talk, and begin the process of challenging and reframing those thoughts. Your future self will thank you for it.

3: Reframing Negative Thoughts

Once you've identified your negative thoughts, it's time to reframe them in a more positive light. In this chapter, we'll provide you with practical exercises and techniques for reframing negative thoughts and beliefs, and replacing them with positive affirmations. Reframing our negative thoughts and beliefs can be a powerful tool for improving our mindset and overall well-being. It's amazing how a simple shift in perspective can help us to see things in a more positive light, and to approach challenges with more confidence and optimism.

In this chapter, we'll provide you with practical exercises and techniques for reframing negative thoughts and beliefs. One effective strategy is to reframe negative thoughts by looking for evidence to the contrary. For example, if you find yourself thinking "I'm not good enough," try to identify examples where you have succeeded or accomplished something in the past. This can help you to see that your negative thought is not entirely accurate or true.

Another effective strategy is to replace negative thoughts with positive affirmations. Affirmations are positive statements that we repeat to ourselves to reinforce positive beliefs and thoughts. For example, if you find yourself thinking "I'll never be able to do this," try replacing that thought with "I am capable and confident, and I can achieve my goals." By repeating these positive affirmations to ourselves, we can begin to rewire our brains to see ourselves in a more positive light.

It's important to remember that reframing negative thoughts and beliefs takes practice and patience. We may not be able to reframe every negative thought immediately, but with consistent effort, we can begin to shift our mindset in a more positive direction.

By reframing our negative thoughts and beliefs, we can begin to see ourselves and the world around us in a more positive light. We can gain more confidence in our abilities, and feel more empowered to pursue our goals and dreams. So, take the time to practice these exercises and techniques for reframing negative thoughts, and watch as your mindset and your life begin to transform in amazing ways.

4: Practicing Gratitude

Gratitude is a powerful tool for shifting your mindset from negative to positive. Let's explore the science behind gratitude, and provide you with practical exercises for cultivating a daily gratitude practice. Practicing gratitude is a powerful way to shift our mindset from negative to positive, and to cultivate more happiness and fulfillment in our lives. Gratitude is all about focusing on the good things in our lives, and appreciating the blessings that we often take for granted.

In this chapter, we'll explore the science behind gratitude, and how it can have a profound impact on our mental and emotional well-being. Research has shown that practicing gratitude can improve our mood, reduce stress, and increase our overall sense of well-being.

One practical exercise for cultivating a daily gratitude practice is to start a gratitude journal. Each day, take a few minutes to write down three things that you're grateful for. These could be anything from small moments of joy, to big accomplishments or blessings in your life. By focusing on the positive and writing it down, we're able to anchor our attention to the good in our lives, and to develop a more positive mindset.

Another practical exercise is to practice gratitude meditation. This involves focusing your attention on the things you're grateful for, and allowing those feelings of gratitude to permeate your body and mind. This can be a great way to start or end your day, and to cultivate a sense of calm and contentment.

It's important to remember that gratitude is a practice, and that it takes consistent effort and intention to develop. But with time and practice, it can become a natural part of our daily routine, and a powerful tool for cultivating a more positive mindset and outlook on life.

By cultivating a daily gratitude practice, we can begin to shift our focus from what's lacking in our lives, to what we're grateful for. We can develop a greater sense of appreciation for the blessings in our lives, and cultivate a more positive and fulfilling mindset. So, take the time to practice gratitude every day, and watch as your mindset and your life begin to transform in amazing ways.

5: Mindfulness and Meditation

Mindfulness and meditation are powerful tools for calming the mind and reducing stress. The benefits of mindfulness and meditation, and provide you with practical exercises for incorporating these practices into your daily life. Mindfulness and meditation are powerful tools for calming the mind and reducing stress. In our busy and hectic lives, it's easy to get caught up in the whirlwind of thoughts and distractions, and to feel overwhelmed and stressed out. But with mindfulness and meditation, we can learn to quiet our minds, focus our attention, and cultivate a sense of inner calm and peace.

The benefits of mindfulness and meditation are numerous. Research has shown that these practices can reduce stress, improve our mood, boost our immune system, and increase our overall sense of well-being. By cultivating a regular mindfulness and meditation practice, we can learn to be more present in the moment, to let go of worries and fears, and to connect more deeply with ourselves and others.

One practical exercise for incorporating mindfulness into your daily life is to practice mindful breathing. This involves focusing your attention on your breath, and allowing your mind to become still and quiet. Simply take a few deep breaths, and then allow your breath to settle into its natural rhythm. As you inhale, focus on the sensation of the breath entering your body. As you exhale, focus on the sensation of the breath leaving your body. If your mind starts to wander, simply notice the thought, and then gently bring your attention back to your breath.

Another practical exercise is to practice a simple meditation. Find a quiet and comfortable space, and sit in a comfortable position. Close your eyes, and focus your attention on your breath. Simply allow your mind to become still and quiet, and allow your thoughts to come and go without judgment. If your mind starts to wander, simply notice the thought, and then gently bring your attention back to your breath.

It's important to remember that mindfulness and meditation are practices, and that it takes consistent effort and intention to develop. But with time and practice, they can become powerful tools for reducing stress, improving our mood, and increasing our overall sense of well-being

6: Visualization Techniques

Visualization is a powerful technique for manifesting your goals and dreams. In we'll provide you with practical exercises for visualizing your ideal future, and creating a vision board to help bring your dreams to life. Visualization is a powerful technique for manifesting our goals and dreams, and bringing our ideal future into reality. It's amazing how the power of our thoughts and imagination can help us to create the life we desire, and to overcome obstacles and challenges along the way.

Now we will provide you with practical exercises for visualizing your ideal future, and creating a vision board to help bring your dreams to life. The first step is to get clear on what you want to manifest in your life. This could be a specific goal or dream, or it could be a more general desire for happiness, fulfillment, and abundance.

Once you've identified your goals and dreams, it's time to start visualizing them. Find a quiet and comfortable space, and allow your mind to become still and quiet. Begin to visualize your ideal future in as much detail as possible. What does it look like? What does it feel like? What are you doing? Who are you with?

It's important to really feel the emotions associated with your visualization, and to allow yourself to experience the joy and excitement of achieving your goals and dreams. This will help to create a powerful and positive energy around your visualization, and to attract more abundance and success into your life.

Another practical exercise is to create a vision board. This involves creating a visual representation of your goals and dreams, using images, words, and symbols that resonate with you. You can create your vision board on a piece of poster board, or on a digital platform like Pinterest.

By regularly visualizing your goals and dreams, and creating a vision board to keep them in front of you, you can create a powerful and positive energy around your desires. This can help you to stay focused and motivated, and to take inspired action towards manifesting your dreams.

So, take the time to practice these visualization exercises, and watch as your goals and dreams begin to take shape in your life. With consistent effort and intention, you can manifest the life you desire, and create a future that is filled with abundance, joy, and fulfillment.

7: The Power of Affirmations

Affirmations are powerful statements that can help you shift your mindset and beliefs. we will now explore the science behind affirmations, and provide you with practical exercises for creating your own positive affirmations. Affirmations are a powerful tool for shifting our mindset and beliefs, and for cultivating a more positive and empowering outlook on life. They are simple yet effective statements that we repeat to ourselves, to reinforce positive beliefs and thoughts.

In this chapter, we'll explore the science behind affirmations, and how they can have a profound impact on our mental and emotional well-being. Research has shown that affirmations can improve our mood, reduce stress, and increase our overall sense of well-being.

One practical exercise for creating your own positive affirmations is to start by identifying the negative thoughts and beliefs that are holding you back. Once you've identified these negative beliefs, you can begin to craft positive affirmations to counteract them. For example, if you find yourself thinking "I'm not good enough," try crafting an affirmation like "I am capable and worthy of success."

It's important to make sure that your affirmations are positive, present-tense statements that resonate with you personally. They should feel authentic and true to you, and should be focused on the kind of person you want to be, or the kind of life you want to create.

Another practical exercise is to repeat your affirmations to yourself regularly, throughout the day. You can write them down on sticky notes and place them around your home or workspace, or you can set a reminder on your phone to repeat them to yourself at specific times of the day.

By incorporating positive affirmations into your daily routine, you can begin to shift your mindset and beliefs in a more positive direction. You can start to see yourself in a more positive light, and believe in your own potential for success and happiness.

So, take the time to practice these exercises for creating and using positive affirmations, and watch as your mindset and your life begin to transform in amazing ways. With consistent effort and intention, you can cultivate a more positive and empowering outlook on life, and create the kind of life you truly desire.

8: Self-Care and Self-Compassion

Self-care and self-compassion are essential components of a positive mindset. Now let's explore the importance of self-care and self-compassion, and provide you with practical strategies for taking care of yourself both physically and emotionally. Self-care and self-compassion are essential components of a positive mindset. In today's fast-paced and stressful world, it's easy to neglect our own physical and emotional well-being. But by making self-care a priority, we can improve our overall health and well-being, and cultivate a more positive and fulfilling life.

In this chapter, we'll explore the importance of self-care and self-compassion, and provide you with practical strategies for taking care of yourself both physically and emotionally. It's important to remember that self-care is not a luxury, but a necessity. It's not selfish to take care of ourselves, but rather an act of self-love and self-respect.

One practical strategy for self-care is to prioritize rest and relaxation. This could involve taking a nap, practicing yoga or meditation, or simply taking a few minutes to breathe deeply and relax. It's important to give ourselves permission to rest and recharge, and to make time for activities that bring us joy and rejuvenation.

Another practical strategy is to practice self-compassion. This involves treating ourselves with kindness and understanding, rather than criticism and judgment. It's important to remember that we're only human, and that we all make mistakes and have flaws. By practicing self-compassion, we can learn to be more accepting of ourselves, and to treat ourselves with the same kindness and compassion that we would offer to a good friend.

It's also important to take care of ourselves physically, by eating well, staying hydrated, and getting regular exercise. These simple yet powerful habits can have a profound impact on our physical and emotional well-being, and can help us to feel more energized and empowered in our daily lives.

By making self-care and self-compassion a priority, we can improve our overall health and well-being, and cultivate a more positive and fulfilling life. So, take the time to practice these strategies for taking care of yourself both physically and emotionally, and watch as your mindset and your life begin to transform in amazing ways. You deserve it!

9: Building a Support System

Having a strong support system is essential for maintaining a positive mindset. the importance of building a support system, and provide you with practical strategies for identifying and cultivating supportive relationships.Building a support system is essential for our emotional well-being, and it can make all the difference in our lives. It's important to surround ourselves with people who uplift us, inspire us, and support us through life's ups and downs. We all need a shoulder to cry on, someone to share our joys and triumphs with, and people who will stand by us no matter what.

Identifying and cultivating supportive relationships can be a challenging task, but it's worth the effort. The first step is to identify the people in your life who bring you joy and positivity. These could be family members, friends, coworkers, or even acquaintances who share similar interests or values. Once you've identified these individuals, it's important to make time to connect with them regularly. This can be as simple as sending a text or making a phone call to check in and see how they're doing.

Building a support system also means being willing to be vulnerable and open with those around you. It can be scary to share our fears, doubts, and struggles with others, but it's important to remember that we're all human and we all go through tough times. By sharing our struggles with trusted friends or family members, we can gain new perspectives and insights, and receive the support and encouragement we need to overcome our challenges.

When building a support system, it's important to be selective about the people you let into your inner circle. Not everyone will be supportive or uplifting, and it's okay to distance yourself from those who bring negativity or toxicity into your life. Instead, focus on cultivating relationships with people who share your values and goals, and who uplift and inspire you to be your best self.

In the end, building a support system is about creating a community of love, kindness, and compassion. It's about surrounding ourselves with people who believe in us, who support our dreams, and who help us to see the beauty and potential in ourselves. So, take the time to identify and cultivate those supportive relationships in your life, and watch as they help you to thrive and grow into the person you were meant to be.

10: Overcoming Obstacles

Obstacles are a natural part of life, but they don't have to hold you back. Obstacles are a natural part of life, and they can be incredibly challenging and frustrating to deal with. It's easy to feel overwhelmed and discouraged when faced with obstacles, and to believe that they are insurmountable barriers to success and happiness.

But the truth is, obstacles don't have to hold you back. In fact, they can be powerful opportunities for growth and learning, and can help you to become stronger, more resilient, and more capable of achieving your goals and dreams.

It's important to remember that everyone faces obstacles in life, and that they are not a reflection of our worth or our abilities. Rather, they are simply challenges that we can choose to overcome with determination, perseverance, and a positive mindset.

One practical strategy for overcoming obstacles is to approach them with a growth mindset. This means viewing obstacles as opportunities for growth and learning, rather than as insurmountable barriers. By adopting a growth mindset, we can cultivate a sense of curiosity and openness, and see obstacles as a chance to learn new skills and develop new strengths.

Another practical strategy is to break down the obstacle into smaller, more manageable steps. By breaking the obstacle into smaller pieces, we can create a clear plan of action, and take consistent and focused steps towards overcoming it.

It's also important to seek support and guidance from others when facing obstacles. Whether it's seeking advice from a mentor, or asking for help from a friend or family member, having a supportive network can be incredibly helpful in navigating challenges and overcoming obstacles.

By approaching obstacles with a positive and growth-oriented mindset, breaking them down into smaller steps, and seeking support and guidance from others, we can overcome even the most challenging obstacles and achieve our goals and dreams. So, don't let obstacles hold you back. Instead, embrace them as opportunities for growth and learning

Chapter 2

SEEDS OF MOTIVATION

If you have you ever found yourself feeling lost or directionless, unsure of what you really want out of life? It's a common feeling, and one that can leave us feeling frustrated, anxious, and unfulfilled. But the good news is, there is a way out of this uncertainty - and it starts with understanding your "why."

Your "why" is your purpose, your reason for being, the thing that drives you and gives your life meaning. It's not just about what you want to do, but why you want to do it. Understanding your why is essential for discovering your passions and setting goals that truly align with your values and aspirations.

But how do you discover your why? It's not always an easy process, and it may take some introspection and soul-searching to uncover it. Here are a few questions to ask yourself that can help:

What brings you joy and fulfillment?

What activities or experiences leave you feeling energized and inspired?

What do you feel most passionate about?

What are your core values, and how do they guide your decisions and actions?

What impact do you want to have on the world, and how can you use your strengths and talents to achieve that impact?

Asking these questions and reflecting on your answers can help you gain a deeper understanding of your purpose and what truly matters to you. It may take time to fully uncover your why, but the journey is worth it.

Once you have a clearer sense of your why, you can use it to guide your goal-setting and decision-making. Your why can serve as a source of motivation and inspiration, reminding you of what you truly care about and what you're working towards. When you have a strong sense of purpose, you're more likely to stay committed to your goals and persist through challenges and setbacks.

So I encourage you to take the time to reflect on your why. It may be a challenging process, but it's one that can lead to greater clarity, fulfillment, and joy in your life. Remember, you are capable of achieving great things, and understanding your why is the first step towards making those things a reality. I encourage you to take the time to reflect on your why. It can be a challenging and emotional process, but it's one that can lead to greater clarity, fulfillment, and joy in your life. It's easy to get caught up in the day-to-day grind, and to lose sight of what truly matters to us. But by understanding our why, we can reconnect with our passions, values, and purpose, and live a life that is truly fulfilling and meaningful.

It's important to remember that you are capable of achieving great things. You have unique talents, gifts, and passions that can make a profound impact on the world around you. But in order to achieve those things, you must first understand your why. What motivates you? What drives you? What brings you joy and fulfillment?

Reflecting on your why can be a challenging and emotional process. It may involve confronting fears and insecurities, or facing difficult truths about yourself and your life. But it's also a process that can be incredibly liberating and empowering. By understanding your why, you can create a clear vision for your life, and take focused and intentional action towards achieving your goals and dreams.

So, take the time to reflect on your why. It may involve journaling, meditating, or seeking guidance from a mentor or therapist. But whatever approach you take, remember that the process is worth it. By understanding your why, you can create a life that is aligned with your deepest values and passions, and experience a greater sense of purpose, joy, and fulfillment. Understanding your why is a powerful and transformative process. When you know what truly motivates you, what you're passionate about, and what brings you the most joy and fulfillment, you can create a life that is aligned with your deepest values and desires.

Living a life that is aligned with your why is incredibly empowering and fulfilling. It means that you are living a life that is authentic to you, rather than one that is defined by the expectations of others or societal norms. It means that you are pursuing your passions and purpose, and making a meaningful impact on the world around you.

When you live a life that is aligned with your why, you experience a greater sense of purpose and fulfillment. You wake up each day with a sense of excitement and enthusiasm, knowing that you are living a life that truly matters to you. You feel a deep sense of connection to your work, your relationships, and your community, and know that you are making a positive impact on the world around you.

But understanding your why isn't always easy. It may require you to confront difficult truths about yourself and your life, or to make challenging decisions about your future. It may involve taking risks and stepping outside of your comfort zone. But the rewards are immeasurable. By understanding your why, you can create a life that is truly fulfilling and meaningful, and experience a greater sense of joy, purpose, and fulfillment.

So, take the time to understand your why. Reflect on your passions, values, and purpose, and create a vision for the kind of life you want to live. Then, take intentional and focused action towards making that vision a reality. It may not always be easy, but the rewards are well worth it. You deserve to live a life that is aligned with your why, and to experience the joy and fulfillment that comes with living a life that truly matters to you.

Chapter 3

OVERCOMING FEAR AND DOUBT

Fear and doubt are powerful emotions that can hold us back from achieving our goals and living the life we truly desire. They can make us feel small, helpless, and overwhelmed, and can prevent us from taking the risks and actions necessary for growth and success.

But the good news is that fear and doubt don't have to hold us back. With the right mindset and strategies, we can learn to overcome these emotions and achieve the success and fulfillment we truly desire.

One practical strategy for overcoming fear and doubt is to face them head-on. This means acknowledging and confronting our fears and doubts, rather than trying to push them aside or ignore them. By facing them directly, we can begin to understand where they are coming from, and develop strategies for overcoming them.

Another practical strategy is to take small, intentional steps towards our goals. This means breaking down our goals into smaller, more manageable steps, and taking focused action towards each one. By taking small steps towards our goals, we can build momentum and confidence, and gradually overcome our fears and doubts.

It's also important to seek support and guidance from others when facing fear and doubt. This could involve seeking advice from a mentor or coach, or simply reaching out to a supportive friend or family member. Having a strong support network can be incredibly helpful in navigating the challenges and uncertainties of life, and can help us to overcome our fears and doubts.

By taking intentional action, facing our fears and doubts head-on, and seeking support from others, we can overcome even the most challenging obstacles and achieve the success and fulfillment we desire. So, don't let fear and doubt hold you back. You are capable of achieving great things, and with the right mindset and strategies, you can overcome any obstacle and live a life that is truly fulfilling and meaningful. t's time to break free from the grip of fear and doubt. Don't let these emotions hold you back from achieving greatness and living a life that is truly fulfilling and meaningful. You are capable of achieving incredible things, and with the right mindset and strategies, you can overcome any obstacle that comes your way.

It's normal to feel afraid or doubtful at times. Life is full of uncertainties and challenges, and it's easy to feel overwhelmed or unsure of ourselves. But it's important to remember that fear and doubt don't have to define us or limit us. We can learn to face them head-on, and develop the resilience and courage necessary to overcome them.

One powerful strategy for overcoming fear and doubt is to cultivate a growth mindset. This means viewing challenges and failures as opportunities for growth and learning, rather than as evidence of our limitations. By adopting a growth mindset, we can learn to see ourselves and our abilities in a more positive light, and take focused and intentional action towards achieving our goals and dreams.

Another practical strategy is to take small, intentional steps towards our goals. By breaking down our goals into smaller, more manageable steps, we can gradually build momentum and confidence, and overcome our fears and doubts. We can also seek support and guidance from others when facing challenges or uncertainties. Whether it's seeking advice from a mentor, or simply reaching out to a supportive friend or family member, having a strong support network can be incredibly helpful in navigating the ups and downs of life. Sometimes our goals can feel overwhelming and out of reach. But the key to achieving them is to take small, intentional steps towards them. By breaking down our goals into smaller, more manageable steps, we can gradually build momentum and confidence, and overcome our fears and doubts.

It's important to remember that every small step we take towards our goals is a step in the right direction. Even if the progress seems slow or incremental, it's still progress. And with each step, we build momentum and confidence, and move closer towards realizing our dreams.

But we don't have to navigate the journey alone. Seeking support and guidance from others can be incredibly helpful in overcoming challenges and uncertainties. Whether it's seeking advice from a mentor, or simply reaching out to a supportive friend or family member, having a strong support network can make all the difference in achieving our goals and dreams.

So, take the first step towards your goals today. Break them down into small, manageable steps, and take intentional action towards each one. And don't forget to seek support and guidance from others along the way. With each step, you'll build momentum and confidence, and move closer towards realizing your dreams

Remember, you are capable of achieving great things. You have unique talents, passions, and strengths that can make a profound impact on the world around you. Don't let fear and doubt hold you back from sharing your gifts with the world. Instead, embrace them as opportunities for growth and learning, and watch as your mindset and your life begin to transform in amazing ways. Take a moment to reflect on your unique talents, passions, and strengths. You have so much to offer the world, and your gifts are waiting to be shared. Don't let fear and doubt hold you back from realizing your full potential. Instead, embrace them as opportunities for growth and learning, and watch as your mindset and your life begin to transform in amazing ways.

It's easy to feel overwhelmed or discouraged when faced with challenges or uncertainties. But it's important to remember that you are capable of achieving great things. You have the power to make a positive impact on the world around you, and to create a life that is truly fulfilling and meaningful.

So, don't let fear and doubt hold you back from sharing your gifts with the world. Embrace them as opportunities for growth and learning, and take intentional action towards achieving your goals and dreams. Whether it's starting a new business, pursuing a creative passion, or making a positive impact in your community, you have the power to create a life that is aligned with your deepest values and desires.

Remember, you are not alone in your journey. Seek support and guidance from others when facing challenges or uncertainties.It's easy to feel like we're on our own when facing challenges or uncertainties. But the truth is, we are not alone in our journey. Seeking support and guidance from others can be incredibly helpful in overcoming obstacles and achieving our goals and dreams.

Whether it's seeking advice from a mentor, or simply reaching out to a supportive friend or family member, having a strong support network can make all the difference. They can offer us encouragement, guidance, and perspective when we need it most.

But seeking support from others can also be difficult. It may require us to be vulnerable and to ask for help, which can be challenging. But it's important to remember that asking for help is not a sign of weakness. It's a sign of strength and courage, and a recognition that we can't do everything on our own.

So, don't be afraid to reach out for help when you need it. Whether you're facing a personal challenge, or struggling to achieve your goals and dreams, seeking support from others can be a powerful tool for growth and success.

Remember, you are not alone in your journey. There are people around you who care about you and want to see you succeed. Don't be afraid to lean on them for support and guidance. Together, you can overcome any obstacle and achieve great things. Whether it's seeking advice from a mentor or coach, or simply reaching out to a supportive friend or family member, having a strong support network can be incredibly helpful in navigating the ups and downs of life.

So, take a deep breath, and believe in yourself and your abilities. You are capable of achieving greatness, and your gifts are waiting to be shared with the world. Embrace the challenges and uncertainties of life as opportunities for growth and learning.

Fear can be a powerful and paralyzing emotion. It can hold us back from pursuing our dreams, trying new things, and living our lives to the fullest. But the truth is, we can get through fear. We can learn to face it head-on, and to take intentional action towards achieving our goals and dreams.

One practical strategy for getting through fear is to confront it directly. This means identifying the source of our fear, and taking intentional steps towards overcoming it. Whether it's seeking support and guidance from others, breaking down our goals into smaller, more manageable steps, or simply taking action despite our fear, confronting our fears can help us to build resilience and courage, and to move closer towards achieving our dreams.

Another strategy is to practice self-compassion. This means being kind and supportive to ourselves, even in the face of fear and uncertainty. It means recognizing that fear is a natural and normal part of the human experience, and that we are not alone in our struggles. By practicing self-compassion, we can learn to be more patient and forgiving with ourselves, and to take intentional action towards our goals and dreams, even when we're feeling afraid.

Ultimately, getting through fear is about taking intentional action towards our goals and dreams, despite the uncertainty and discomfort that may come with it. It's about recognizing that fear is a natural part of the human experience, and that we have the power to overcome it. So, take a deep breath, and believe in yourself and your abilities. We can learn to overcome our fears and take intentional action towards achieving our goals and dreams.

One practical strategy for fighting through fear is to practice mindfulness. This means being present in the moment and observing our thoughts and emotions without judgment. By practicing mindfulness, we can learn to recognize when fear is arising, and to respond to it in a more intentional and thoughtful way.

Another strategy is to surround ourselves with supportive and encouraging people. Having a strong support network can provide us with the encouragement and motivation we need to push through our fears and pursue our dreams. Whether it's seeking advice from a mentor, or simply reaching out to a supportive friend or family member, having people around us who believe in us can make all the difference.

It's also important to take small, intentional steps towards our goals. By breaking down our goals into smaller, more manageable steps, we can gradually build momentum and confidence, and overcome our fears and doubts. We can also celebrate our successes along the way, no matter how small they may be, to build our confidence and motivation.

Ultimately, fighting through fear is about taking intentional action towards our goals and dreams, even when it's uncomfortable or scary

Chapter 4

FINDING PURPOSE AND MEANING

At some point in our lives, we may find ourselves asking the question, "What is my purpose?" It's a question that can stir up feelings of uncertainty, confusion, and even despair. But the good news is that finding purpose and meaning in our lives is possible, and it can bring us a sense of fulfillment, joy, and satisfaction beyond measure.

One practical strategy for finding purpose and meaning is to explore our passions and interests. What are the things that light us up and make us feel alive? What brings us joy and a sense of fulfillment? By identifying our passions and interests, we can begin to explore how we can use them to create a life that is aligned with our deepest values and desires.

Another strategy is to seek out opportunities for growth and learning. Whether it's taking a class, learning a new skill, or pursuing a personal goal, seeking out opportunities for growth and learning can help us to discover new passions and interests, and to find deeper meaning and purpose in our lives.

It's also important to surround ourselves with people and experiences that bring us joy and fulfillment. Whether it's spending time with loved ones, volunteering for a cause we believe in, or pursuing a creative passion, finding ways to incorporate joy and fulfillment into our lives can help us to feel more connected and purposeful.

Ultimately, finding purpose and meaning in our lives is about understanding what truly matters to us, and using that understanding to guide our decisions and actions. It's about aligning our lives with our deepest values and passions, and creating a life that is fulfilling, meaningful, and true to who we are.

Take the time to explore your passions and interests, seek out opportunities for growth and learning, and surround yourself with people and experiences that bring you joy and fulfillment. By doing so, you'll be one step closer to discovering your purpose and living a life that is truly fulfilling and meaningful. Finding meaning in our lives is something that many of us strive for. It's a journey that can be filled with ups and downs, but it's also one that can bring us a sense of purpose, fulfillment, and joy beyond measure.

One practical strategy for finding meaning is to explore our passions and interests. What are the things that light us up and make us feel alive? What brings us joy and a sense of fulfillment? By identifying our passions and interests, we can begin to explore how we can use them to create a life that is aligned with our deepest values and desires.

Another strategy is to seek out opportunities for growth and learning. Whether it's taking a class, learning a new skill, or pursuing a personal goal, seeking out opportunities for growth and learning can help us to discover new passions and interests, and to find deeper meaning and purpose in our lives.

It's also important to surround ourselves with people and experiences that bring us joy and fulfillment. Whether it's spending time with loved ones, volunteering for a cause we believe in, or pursuing a creative passion, finding ways to incorporate joy and fulfillment into our lives can help us to feel more connected and purposeful.

Ultimately, finding meaning in our lives is about understanding what truly matters to us, and using that understanding to guide our decisions and actions. It's about aligning our lives with our deepest values and passions, and creating a life that is fulfilling, meaningful, and true to who we are.

So, take the time to explore your passions and interests, seek out opportunities for growth and learning, and surround yourself with people and experiences that bring you joy and fulfillment. By doing so, you'll be one step closer to discovering your purpose and living a life that is truly fulfilling and meaningful. Finding our purpose in life can be a daunting task, one that can leave us feeling lost, confused, and uncertain. But it's also a journey that can bring us a sense of clarity, fulfillment, and joy beyond measure.

One practical strategy for finding our purpose is to reflect on our values and beliefs. What are the things that matter most to us? What do we believe in? By identifying our values and beliefs, we can begin to explore how we can use them to create a life that is aligned with our deepest desires.

Another strategy is to explore our passions and interests. What are the things that we love to do? What brings us joy and a sense of fulfillment? By identifying our passions and interests, we can begin to explore how we can use them to create a life that is meaningful and purposeful.

It's also important to seek out opportunities for growth and learning. Whether it's taking a class, learning a new skill, or pursuing a personal goal, seeking out opportunities for growth and learning can help us to discover new passions and interests, and to find deeper meaning and purpose in our lives.

Ultimately, finding our purpose in life is about understanding who we are, what we believe in, and what truly matters to us. It's about aligning our lives with our deepest desires and passions, and creating a life that is fulfilling, meaningful, and true to who we are.

So, take the time to reflect on your values and beliefs, explore your passions and interests, and seek out opportunities for growth and learning. By doing so, you'll be one step closer to discovering your purpose. Our core beliefs are the fundamental ideas and values that shape our perceptions of ourselves and the world around us. They are the lens through which we interpret our experiences, and they can have a powerful impact on our thoughts, emotions, and behaviors.

Identifying our core beliefs can be a challenging process,

but it's also a crucial one. By understanding our core beliefs, we can begin to challenge any negative or limiting beliefs that may be holding us back, and replace them with more positive and empowering ones.

One practical strategy for identifying our core beliefs is to reflect on our past experiences and how they have shaped our perceptions of ourselves and the world around us. What messages did we receive from our parents, teachers, or other authority figures growing up? What events or experiences have had the greatest impact on our sense of self and our beliefs about the world?

Another strategy is to pay attention to our thoughts and emotions. What do we tell ourselves when we experience a setback or failure? What are our automatic thoughts and assumptions about ourselves and others? By becoming more aware of our thoughts and emotions, we can begin to identify any negative or limiting beliefs that may be holding us back.

Ultimately, challenging and replacing our core beliefs is about recognizing that we have the power to shape our perceptions of ourselves and the world around us. It's about choosing to believe in ourselves and our abilities, even in the face of adversity or uncertainty. It's about embracing a growth mindset, and recognizing that we have the capacity to learn, grow, and change throughout our lives.

So, take the time to reflect on your past experiences and your thoughts and emotions. Identify any negative or limiting core beliefs that may be holding you back, and challenge them with positive and empowering ones. an addiction even one that you dont realize is there can counter these actions. Fighting our addictions can be one of the most challenging and emotional journeys we can undertake. Addiction can take hold of our lives, leaving us feeling powerless and helpless. But it's important to remember that we are not alone, and that with the right mindset, strategies, and support, we can overcome our addictions and reclaim our lives.

One practical strategy for fighting our addictions is to develop a support network. This can include family, friends, support groups, and professionals. Having people around us who believe in us and our ability to overcome our addiction can provide us with the motivation and encouragement we need to keep going.

Another strategy is to practice self-care and self-compassion. Addiction can be a painful and difficult experience, and it's important to take care of ourselves both physically and emotionally. This can include engaging in activities that bring us joy and fulfillment, such as exercise or creative pursuits, and seeking professional help if necessary.

It's also important to understand the root causes of our addiction. Addiction is often a symptom of underlying emotional or psychological issues, such as trauma or anxiety. By addressing these issues through therapy or other interventions, we can begin to heal and move towards a more positive and fulfilling life.

Ultimately, fighting our addictions is about making a commitment to ourselves and our well-being. It's about recognizing that we are worthy of a life free from addiction, and taking intentional action towards that goal. It's about embracing a growth mindset, and recognizing that we have the power to learn, grow, and change throughout our lives.

So, take the time to develop a support network, practice self-care and self-compassion, and address the underlying causes of your addiction. Remember, you are not alone, and you have the power to overcome your addiction and reclaim your life. Restructuring our lives can be a daunting and emotional process.

It can mean making significant changes, letting go of old patterns, and embracing new opportunities. But it's also a journey that can bring us a greater sense of purpose, fulfillment, and joy.

One practical strategy for restructuring our lives is to identify our priorities and values. What matters most to us? What are our deepest desires and dreams? By identifying our priorities and values, we can begin to align our lives with what truly matters to us, and create a sense of purpose and meaning.

Another strategy is to identify areas of our lives that are not serving us well, and take intentional action to change them. This can mean setting boundaries, letting go of toxic relationships or behaviors, and creating new habits and routines that support our goals and values.

It's also important to practice self-compassion and give ourselves permission to make mistakes and learn from them. Restructuring our lives can be a challenging process, and it's important to be patient and kind to ourselves as we navigate the ups and downs.

Ultimately, restructuring our lives is about embracing change and growth. It's about recognizing that we have the power to shape our lives in a way that is fulfilling and meaningful. It's about embracing a growth mindset, and recognizing that we have the capacity to learn, grow, and change throughout our lives.

So, take the time to identify your priorities and values, and take intentional action towards creating a life that is aligned with what matters most to you. Remember, restructuring your life is a journey, and it's one that can bring you a greater sense of purpose, fulfillment, and joy.

Chapter 5

THE IMPORTANCE OF SELF-REFLECTION

Have you ever set a goal, only to find yourself losing motivation and making little progress towards it? It's a frustrating feeling, but it's one that can be avoided with the power of SMART goals.

SMART goals are specific, measurable, achievable, relevant, and time-bound. By setting goals that meet these criteria, you can ensure that they are clear, actionable, and aligned with your values and aspirations.

Setting SMART goals can be a powerful tool for achieving your dreams and creating the life you want. By breaking down your goals into specific, achievable steps, you can stay focused and motivated, even when the road gets tough.

But setting SMART goals is more than just a process - it's an emotional journey. It requires vulnerability, self-reflection, and a willingness to confront your fears and limitations. It can be scary to set ambitious goals, knowing that there's a chance you may fail.

But the truth is, the only way to achieve great things is to take risks and push yourself outside of your comfort zone.

The key to setting SMART goals is to start small and build momentum. Focus on one goal at a time, and break it down into specific, measurable steps. Celebrate your progress along the way, and don't be afraid to ask for help or support when you need it.

Remember, setting SMART goals is not just about achieving external success - it's also about cultivating a growth mindset and a sense of purpose and fulfillment in your life. When you set goals that align with your values and aspirations, you create a roadmap for living the life you truly want.

So I encourage you to take the time to set SMART goals for yourself. Embrace the emotional journey of self-reflection and vulnerability, and don't be afraid to dream big. You are capable of achieving great things, and setting SMART goals is the first step towards making those things a reality.

Setting SMART goals can be a powerful strategy for achieving our dreams and making positive changes in our lives. It can provide us with clarity, focus, and motivation, and help us to create a life that is aligned with our deepest desires.

One practical strategy for setting SMART goals is to identify our specific, measurable, achievable, relevant, and time-bound goals. By setting goals that are specific, we can create a clear and defined target for ourselves. By making our goals measurable, we can track our progress and celebrate our successes. By setting goals that are achievable, we can avoid feeling overwhelmed or discouraged. By setting goals that are relevant, we can ensure that they are aligned with our priorities and values. And by setting goals that are time-bound, we can create a sense of urgency and motivation to take action.

It's also important to stay focused on our goals and to stay motivated. This can include creating a plan of action, breaking down our goals into smaller, more manageable steps, and celebrating our successes along the way.

Ultimately, setting SMART goals is about taking intentional action towards creating a life that is aligned with our deepest desires and values. It's about embracing a growth mindset, and recognizing that we have the power to learn, grow, and change throughout our lives.

So, take the time to identify your SMART goals, and take intentional action towards achieving them. Remember, you are capable of achieving great things, and setting SMART goals is one powerful strategy for making positive changes in your life. Setting SMART goals can be a powerful tool for achieving our dreams and making positive changes in our lives. SMART goals are specific, measurable, achievable, relevant, and time-bound goals that help us to create a clear and defined target for ourselves.

Here is a breakdown of what each element of a SMART goal means:

Specific: A specific goal is clear and well-defined, with a specific outcome in mind. It answers the questions: What exactly do I want to achieve? Why is this goal important to me?

Measurable: A measurable goal is one that can be tracked and quantified, so that progress can be monitored and success can be celebrated. It answers the question: How will I know when I have achieved my goal?

Achievable: An achievable goal is one that is realistic and attainable, given the resources and time available. It answers the question: Is this goal realistic for me to achieve?

Relevant: A relevant goal is one that is aligned with our priorities, values, and larger vision for our lives. It answers the question: Is this goal relevant to my overall life purpose and vision?

Time-bound: A time-bound goal is one that has a specific deadline or timeframe for completion. It creates a sense of urgency and motivation to take action, and helps us to stay focused and accountable.

By setting SMART goals, we can create a clear and defined target for ourselves, and take intentional action towards achieving our dreams and desires. It's an emotional journey, as we work towards creating a life that is aligned with our deepest values and passions. But with perseverance and dedication, we can achieve great things and create a life that is fulfilling and meaningful.

Chapter 6

BUILDING RESILIENCE

Have you ever felt like you weren't good enough, smart enough, or talented enough to achieve your dreams? It's a painful feeling, and one that can hold you back from pursuing your passions and living your best life. But the truth is, you are capable of achieving great things - and it all starts with developing a growth mindset.

A growth mindset is the belief that your abilities and talents can be developed through hard work, dedication, and perseverance. It's the idea that you are not limited by your natural talents or intelligence, but rather by your effort and attitude.

Developing a growth mindset can be a powerful tool for overcoming obstacles, achieving your goals, and living a more fulfilling life. By embracing the idea that you can always learn and grow, you open yourself up to new opportunities and possibilities.

But developing a growth mindset is not always easy. It requires a willingness to embrace failure and setbacks as opportunities for learning and growth. It requires a willingness to challenge yourself and step outside of your comfort zone. It requires a willingness to believe in yourself, even when others doubt you.

The journey towards a growth mindset is an emotional one, filled with ups and downs, triumphs and setbacks. But every time you face a challenge with a growth mindset, you become stronger and more resilient.

So I encourage you to embrace the journey towards a growth mindset. Believe in yourself and your ability to learn and grow. Celebrate your successes, but also embrace your failures as opportunities for growth. Surround yourself with positivity and support, and don't be afraid to ask for help when you need it.

Remember, developing a growth mindset is not just about achieving external success - it's about cultivating a sense of purpose and fulfillment in your life. When you approach challenges with a growth mindset, you become more confident, more resilient, and more fulfilled. Developing a growth mindset can be a transformative journey, as it empowers us to approach challenges with confidence, resilience, and fulfillment. It's an emotional journey that requires us to let go of limiting beliefs and embrace new possibilities.

Remember, developing a growth mindset is not just about achieving external success. It's about cultivating a deeper sense of purpose and fulfillment in our lives. It's about recognizing our own worth and potential, and taking intentional action towards achieving our dreams and desires.

When we approach challenges with a growth mindset, we become more confident in our abilities and more resilient in the face of setbacks. We begin to see failures and obstacles as opportunities for growth and learning, rather than as sources of shame or self-doubt.

Ultimately, developing a growth mindset is about creating a life that is aligned with our deepest values and passions. It's about embracing a sense of purpose and fulfillment, and recognizing that we have the power to shape our lives in meaningful and rewarding ways.

So, embrace the journey of developing a growth mindset, and approach every challenge with a sense of possibility and opportunity. Having a growth mindset means believing that our abilities and intelligence can be developed through hard work, dedication, and perseverance. It's an emotional journey that requires us to let go of limiting beliefs and embrace new possibilities.

Here are some key characteristics of a growth mindset:

Embracing challenges: People with a growth mindset see challenges as opportunities for growth and learning, and they are not afraid to step outside of their comfort zones.

Persistence and effort: People with a growth mindset understand that achieving success requires effort and persistence, and they are willing to put in the work to achieve their goals.

Learning from feedback: People with a growth mindset see feedback as an opportunity for learning and improvement, and they use it to guide their actions and decisions.

Embracing failure: People with a growth mindset see failure as a natural part of the learning process, and they use it as an opportunity to reflect, learn, and grow.

Celebrating others' success: People with a growth mindset celebrate the success of others, and they see it as evidence that success is attainable with hard work and dedication.

Ultimately, developing a growth mindset is about creating a life that is aligned with our deepest values and passions. It's about recognizing our own worth and potential, and taking intentional action towards achieving our dreams and desires.

So, embrace the journey of developing a growth mindset, and approach every challenge with a sense of possibility and opportunity.Having a growth mindset means believing that our abilities and intelligence can be developed through hard work, dedication, and perseverance. It's an emotional journey that requires us to let go of limiting beliefs and embrace new possibilities.

Here are some key characteristics of a growth mindset:

Embracing challenges: People with a growth mindset see challenges as opportunities for growth and learning, and they are not afraid to step outside of their comfort zones.

Persistence and effort: People with a growth mindset understand that achieving success requires effort and persistence, and they are willing to put in the work to achieve their goals.

Learning from feedback: People with a growth mindset see feedback as an opportunity for learning and improvement, and they use it to guide their actions and decisions.

Embracing failure: People with a growth mindset see failure as a natural part of the learning process, and they use it as an opportunity to reflect, learn, and grow.

Celebrating others' success: People with a growth mindset celebrate the success of others, and they see it as evidence that success is attainable with hard work and dedication.

Ultimately, developing a growth mindset is about creating a life that is aligned with our deepest values and passions. It's about recognizing our own worth and potential, and taking intentional action towards achieving our dreams and desires.

So, embrace the journey of developing a growth mindset, and approach every challenge with a sense of possibility and opportunity. Having a growth mindset means believing that our abilities and intelligence can be developed through hard work, dedication, and perseverance. It's an emotional journey that requires us to let go of limiting beliefs and embrace new possibilities.

Here are some key characteristics of a growth mindset:

Embracing challenges: People with a growth mindset see challenges as opportunities for growth and learning, and they are not afraid to step outside of their comfort zones.

Persistence and effort: People with a growth mindset understand that achieving success requires effort and persistence, and they are willing to put in the work to achieve their goals.

Learning from feedback: People with a growth mindset see feedback as an opportunity for learning and improvement, and they use it to guide their actions and decisions.

Embracing failure: People with a growth mindset see failure as a natural part of the learning process, and they use it as an opportunity to reflect, learn, and grow.

Celebrating others' success: People with a growth mindset celebrate the success of others, and they see it as evidence that success is attainable with hard work and dedication.

Ultimately, developing a growth mindset is about creating a life that is aligned with our deepest values and passions. It's about recognizing our own worth and potential, and taking intentional action towards achieving our dreams and desires.

So, embrace the journey of developing a growth mindset, and approach every challenge with a sense of possibility and opportunity.

Having a growth mindset means believing that our abilities and intelligence can be developed through hard work, dedication, and perseverance. It's an emotional journey that requires us to let go of limiting beliefs and embrace new possibilities.

Here are some key characteristics of a growth mindset:

Embracing challenges: People with a growth mindset see challenges as opportunities for growth and learning, and they are not afraid to step outside of their comfort zones. Embracing challenges is an emotional journey that requires us to step outside of our comfort zones and push ourselves to new heights. It can be scary and intimidating, but it's also incredibly rewarding and fulfilling.

People with a growth mindset understand that challenges are not obstacles to be feared, but rather opportunities for growth and learning. They see each challenge as a chance to push themselves further and to develop new skills and abilities.

When we embrace challenges with a growth mindset, we open ourselves up to new experiences and possibilities. We become more confident in our abilities, and we begin to see ourselves as capable of achieving great things.

So, don't be afraid to embrace challenges and step outside of your comfort zone. Remember, each challenge is an opportunity for growth and learning, and with a growth mindset, you can achieve great things and create a life that is truly fulfilling and meaningful.

Persistence and effort: People with a growth mindset understand that achieving success requires effort and persistence, and they are willing to put in the work to achieve their goals. Persistence and effort are key components of developing a growth mindset, as they require us to work hard and stay committed to our goals even when things get tough. It can be challenging and exhausting at times, but it's also incredibly empowering and rewarding.

People with a growth mindset understand that achieving success requires effort and persistence. They are willing to put in the work and to stay committed to their goals, even when faced with obstacles or setbacks. They believe in their own abilities and are willing to work hard to achieve their dreams and desires.

When we embrace persistence and effort with a growth mindset, we develop a sense of resilience and determination that can carry us through even the most difficult of challenges. We become more confident in our abilities and more resilient in the face of setbacks.

So, don't be afraid to put in the effort and stay persistent in pursuing your goals. Remember, with a growth mindset, you can achieve great things and create a life that is truly fulfilling and meaningful.

Learning from feedback: People with a growth mindset see feedback as an opportunity for learning and improvement, and they use it to guide their actions and decisions. Learning from feedback is an emotional journey that requires us to embrace vulnerability and openness to new perspectives. It can be challenging to receive feedback, but it's also incredibly valuable and necessary for growth and improvement.

People with a growth mindset see feedback as an opportunity for learning and improvement. They understand that feedback, even if it's negative, can be used to guide their actions and decisions. They approach feedback with openness and a willingness to learn, even if it means facing uncomfortable truths about themselves.

When we embrace feedback with a growth mindset, we become more self-aware and more open to new perspectives. We develop a sense of humility and a willingness to improve, even if it means facing criticism or admitting our own mistakes.

So, don't be afraid to embrace feedback and use it to guide your actions and decisions. Remember, with a growth mindset, you can learn and improve from any feedback, even if it's difficult to receive.

Embracing failure: People with a growth mindset see failure as a natural part of the learning process, and they use it as an opportunity to reflect, learn, and grow. Embracing failure is an emotional journey that requires us to let go of our fear of failure and to embrace the lessons that come from it. It can be difficult to face failure, but it's also incredibly liberating and empowering.

People with a growth mindset see failure as a natural part of the learning process. They understand that failure is not a reflection of their worth or abilities, but rather an opportunity to reflect, learn, and grow. They approach failure with curiosity and a willingness to learn from their mistakes.

When we embrace failure with a growth mindset, we become more resilient and more adaptable. We develop a sense of courage and a willingness to take risks, even if it means facing the possibility of failure.

So, don't be afraid to embrace failure and to use it as an opportunity to reflect, learn, and grow. Remember, with a growth mindset, failure is not a setback, but rather a necessary step towards success and fulfillment.

Celebrating others' success: People with a growth mindset

celebrate the success of others, and they see it as evidence that success is attainable with hard work and dedication. Celebrating others' success is an emotional journey that requires us to let go of our own insecurities and to embrace the success of those around us. It can be challenging to see others succeed, but it's also incredibly inspiring and motivating.

People with a growth mindset celebrate the success of others. They see it as evidence that success is attainable with hard work and dedication, and they use it as a source of inspiration for their own growth and development. They approach the success of others with a sense of generosity and gratitude, rather than envy or competition.

When we celebrate the success of others with a growth mindset, we become more supportive and more empathetic. We develop a sense of gratitude and a willingness to learn from the successes of others, rather than feeling threatened or intimidated by them.

So, don't be afraid to celebrate the success of others and to use it as a source of inspiration for your own growth and development. Remember, with a growth mindset, the success of others is not a threat, but rather a celebration of the limitless potential within us all.

Ultimately, developing a growth mindset is about creating a life that is aligned with our deepest values and passions. It's about recognizing our own worth and potential, and taking intentional action towards achieving our dreams and desires.

So, embrace the journey of developing a growth mindset, and approach every challenge with a sense of possibility and opportunity.

Chapter 7

CULTIVATING POSITIVE HABITS

Have you ever set a goal for yourself, only to find yourself struggling to make progress towards it? It's a frustrating feeling, but the good news is that there's a way to make achieving your goals easier - and it starts with creating habits that support them.

Habits are powerful tools that can either help or hinder our progress towards our goals. When we create habits that support our goals, we make it easier to take consistent action and make progress towards what we want.

But creating new habits is not always easy. It requires a willingness to step out of your comfort zone and try new things. It requires a willingness to be patient and persistent, even when results don't come right away.

The key to creating habits that support your goals is to start small and build momentum. Focus on one habit at a time, and make it specific, measurable, and achievable. Celebrate your progress along the way, and don't be too hard on yourself when you slip up.

Creating habits that support your goals is an emotional journey, filled with ups and downs, triumphs and setbacks. But every time you take action towards your goals, you become stronger and more confident.

So I encourage you to start creating habits that support your goals today. Take small, consistent steps towards what you want, and celebrate your progress along the way. Surround yourself with positivity and support, and don't be afraid to ask for help when you need it. Remember, creating habits that support your goals is not just about achieving external success - it's about cultivating a sense of purpose and fulfillment in your life. When you create habits that align with your values and aspirations, you create a foundation for living the life you truly want. Positive aspirations are the emotional fuel that drives us towards our goals and dreams. They are the hopes, dreams, and desires that inspire us to take action and to strive for something greater.

Positive aspirations can take many forms, from career goals and personal achievements to relationships and spiritual growth. They are a reflection of our deepest values and passions, and they give us a sense of purpose and meaning in our lives.

When we focus on our positive aspirations with a growth mindset, we become more motivated and more resilient. We develop a sense of clarity and direction, and we begin to see our dreams and desires as achievable and within reach.

So, don't be afraid to embrace your positive aspirations and to use them as a source of motivation and inspiration. Remember, with a growth mindset, anything is possible, and your positive aspirations can lead you to a life of fulfillment and joy. Achieving spiritual growth is an emotional journey that requires us to cultivate a deep sense of connection and purpose. It can be challenging to find spiritual fulfillment, but it's also incredibly rewarding and fulfilling.

To achieve spiritual growth, we must first take the time to connect with our inner selves and to cultivate a sense of mindfulness and presence. This can be done through meditation, prayer, or simply taking the time to reflect and connect with nature.

We must also cultivate a sense of compassion and empathy towards ourselves and others. This can be done by practicing forgiveness, gratitude, and generosity, and by seeking to understand and connect with those around us.

Finally, we must live our lives with intention and purpose. This means aligning our actions and decisions with our deepest values and passions, and working towards a greater sense of meaning and fulfillment in our lives.

When we embrace spiritual growth with a growth mindset, we become more grounded, more compassionate, and more connected to ourselves and those around us. We develop a sense of purpose and fulfillment that transcends the material world, and we begin to see life in a more meaningful and purposeful way.

So, don't be afraid to embrace spiritual growth and to use it as a source of connection and purpose in your life. Remember, with a growth mindset, spiritual fulfillment is not a far-off goal, but rather a daily practice. Becoming more grounded is an emotional journey that requires us to connect with our inner selves and to cultivate a sense of mindfulness and presence. It can be challenging to feel grounded, but it's also incredibly liberating and empowering.

To become more grounded, we must first take the time to connect with our bodies and our surroundings. This can be done through practices like yoga, meditation, or simply taking a walk in nature.

We must also cultivate a sense of gratitude and appreciation for the present moment. This means learning to let go of our worries and anxieties about the future, and to embrace the beauty and richness of the present moment.

Finally, we must live our lives with intention and purpose. This means aligning our actions and decisions with our deepest values and passions, and working towards a greater sense of meaning and fulfillment in our lives.

When we embrace grounding with a growth mindset, we become more centered, more present, and more connected to ourselves and those around us. We develop a sense of inner peace and stability that transcends the chaos and uncertainty of the external world, and we begin to see life in a more calm and centered way.

So, don't be afraid to embrace grounding and to use it as a source of inner peace and stability in your life. Embracing inner peace is an emotional journey that requires us to connect with our inner selves and to cultivate a sense of mindfulness and presence. It can be challenging to find inner peace, but it's also incredibly liberating and empowering.

To embrace inner peace, we must first take the time to quiet our minds and to connect with our breath. This can be done through practices like meditation, yoga, or simply taking a few deep breaths.

We must also cultivate a sense of gratitude and appreciation for the present moment. This means learning to let go of our worries and anxieties about the past or future, and to embrace the beauty and richness of the present moment.

Finally, we must live our lives with intention and purpose. This means aligning our actions and decisions with our deepest values and passions, and working towards a greater sense of meaning and fulfillment in our lives.

When we embrace inner peace with a growth mindset, we become more centered, more present, and more connected to ourselves and those around us. We develop a sense of inner peace and tranquility that transcends the chaos and uncertainty of the external world, and we begin to see life in a more calm and peaceful way.

So, don't be afraid to embrace inner peace and to use it as a source of inner strength and tranquility in your life. Having a spiritual mantra can be a powerful tool for connecting with our inner selves and cultivating a sense of mindfulness and presence. It can be a way to ground ourselves in times of stress and uncertainty, and to remind ourselves of our deepest values and passions.

Your spiritual mantra can be anything that resonates with you, whether it's a word, a phrase, or a simple statement of intention. It should be something that speaks to your heart and helps you to connect with your deepest sense of purpose and meaning.

When you repeat your spiritual mantra with a growth mindset, you can feel a deep sense of peace and tranquility wash over you. You become more centered, more present, and more connected to yourself and the world around you.

So, take some time to find your spiritual mantra and to repeat it daily with intention and purpose. Allow it to ground you and to connect you with your deepest sense of self and purpose

Chapter 8

CREATING A VISION FOR YOUR LIFE

Have you ever felt like you were stuck in a rut, unable to make progress towards your goals? It's a frustrating feeling, but the good news is that there's a way out of it - and it starts with creating habits that support your goals.

Habits are powerful tools that can either help or hinder our progress towards what we want. When we create habits that support our goals, we make it easier to take consistent action and make progress towards what we want.

But creating new habits is not always easy. It requires a willingness to step out of your comfort zone and try new things. It requires a willingness to be patient and persistent, even when results don't come right away.

The key to creating habits that support your goals is to start small and build momentum. Focus on one habit at a time, and make it specific, measurable, and achievable. Celebrate your progress along the way, and don't be too hard on yourself when you slip up.

Creating habits that support your goals is an emotional journey, filled with ups and downs, triumphs and setbacks. But every time you take action towards your goals, you become stronger and more confident.

So I encourage you to start creating habits that support your goals today. Take small, consistent steps towards what you want, and celebrate your progress along the way. Surround yourself with positivity and support, and don't be afraid to ask for help when you need it.

Remember, creating habits that support your goals is not just about achieving external success - it's about cultivating a sense of purpose and fulfillment in your life. When you create habits that align with your values and aspirations, you create a foundation for living the life you truly want. Vision boards are a powerful tool for manifesting your goals and dreams. There are many different kinds of vision boards that you can create, each with its own unique focus and purpose.

One type of vision board is a visual representation of your goals and aspirations. This can include images and words that represent the things that you want to achieve, such as a dream job, a new home, or a fulfilling relationship. Creating this type of vision board can help you to stay focused on your goals and to manifest them into your reality. this is called manifestation. Creating a vision board of your goals and aspirations can be an incredibly inspiring and uplifting experience. By filling your board with images and words that represent the things that you want to achieve, you can tap into the power of visualization and begin to manifest your dreams into reality.

As you create your vision board, allow yourself to dream big and to imagine a life that is filled with joy, purpose, and fulfillment. Let your imagination run wild, and don't hold back on the things that you truly desire.

As you add each image or word to your board, allow yourself to feel the excitement and energy that comes with envisioning your future. Allow yourself to feel the emotions that come with achieving your goals and living the life that you truly desire.

Remember, with a growth mindset, anything is possible. By creating a vision board of your goals and aspirations, you can stay focused on what truly matters, and take intentional steps towards creating a life that is filled with purpose, joy, and fulfillment.

So, take some time to create your vision board today, and allow yourself to tap into the power of visualization and manifestation.

Another type of vision board is a gratitude board, which is a visual representation of the things that you are grateful for in your life. This can include images and words that represent the people, places, and experiences that bring you joy and fulfillment. Creating this type of vision board can help you to cultivate a sense of gratitude and appreciation for the present moment. Creating a gratitude board can be a truly heartwarming and transformative experience. By filling your board with images and words that represent the things that you are grateful for in your life, you can cultivate a deeper sense of gratitude and appreciation for the present moment.

As you create your gratitude board, allow yourself to reflect on the people, places, and experiences that bring you joy and fulfillment. Let yourself feel the emotions that come with experiencing these moments of joy and gratitude.

Each image or word that you add to your board is a reminder of the abundance and blessings that surround you every day. As you look at your board, allow yourself to feel the warmth and love that comes with gratitude, and know that you are truly blessed.

Remember, with a growth mindset, even the smallest things can bring great joy and fulfillment. By creating a gratitude board, you can cultivate a deep sense of appreciation for the present moment, and embrace all of the blessings that life has to offer. So, take some time to create your gratitude board today, and allow yourself to bask in the warmth and love of gratitude.

A third type of vision board is a mindfulness board, which is a visual representation of the things that help you to feel centered and present in the moment. This can include images and words that represent practices like meditation, yoga, or spending time in nature. Creating this type of vision board can help you to cultivate a sense of mindfulness and presence in your daily life. Creating a mindfulness board can be a truly transformative and grounding experience. By filling your board with images and words that represent the things that help you to feel centered and present in the moment, you can cultivate a deeper sense of mindfulness and presence in your daily life.

As you create your mindfulness board, allow yourself to reflect on the practices and experiences that bring you a sense of calm and inner peace. Let yourself feel the emotions that come with experiencing these moments of mindfulness and presence.

Each image or word that you add to your board is a reminder of the importance of taking time for yourself and staying present in the moment. As you look at your board, allow yourself to feel the peace and serenity that comes with mindfulness, and know that you are truly taking care of yourself.

Remember, with a growth mindset, taking time for yourself and practicing mindfulness can have a profound impact on your mental and emotional wellbeing. By creating a mindfulness board, you can cultivate a deep sense of presence and peace in your daily life, and stay connected to the things that truly matter. So, take some time to create your mindfulness board today, and allow yourself to bask in the calm and serenity of mindfulness.

No matter what type of vision board you create, remember to approach it with a growth mindset. Allow yourself to dream big, to embrace the power of visualization, and to take intentional steps towards manifesting your goals and dreams. Remember, with a growth mindset, your vision board can be a powerful tool for creating a life of greater purpose, fulfillment, and joy. Approaching your vision board with a growth mindset can be a truly transformative and inspiring experience. Allow yourself to dream big, to embrace the power of visualization, and to take intentional steps towards manifesting your goals and dreams.

Remember, with a growth mindset, anything is possible. Your vision board can be a powerful tool for creating a life of greater purpose, fulfillment, and joy. As you create your board, allow yourself to dream big, to embrace your innermost passions and desires, and to visualize the life that you truly want to live.

With each image or word that you add to your board, feel the power of manifestation at work. Allow yourself to connect with the energy and vibration of your dreams and aspirations, and know that they are already coming to life.

Remember, a growth mindset is all about taking intentional action towards your goals and dreams. With your vision board as your guide, you can take inspired action each day, and watch as your dreams begin to unfold before your very eyes.

So, go ahead and create your vision board with confidence and excitement. Allow yourself to embrace the power of visualization and manifestation, and watch as your dreams become your reality. With a growth mindset, anything is possible, and the sky truly is the limit!

Chapter 9

THE ROLE OF PASSION IN MOTIVATION

Have you ever felt uninspired, like you're stuck in a rut and can't find the motivation to pursue your passions? It's a frustrating feeling, but the good news is that inspiration can be found in the most unexpected places - even in your daily life.

Finding inspiration in daily life is an emotional journey, one that requires a willingness to be present and open to the world around you. It's about finding beauty in the ordinary, and seeing the extraordinary in the mundane.

One way to find inspiration in daily life is to practice gratitude. Take the time to appreciate the small things in your life, like the warmth of the sun on your skin or the taste of your favorite food. By focusing on what you have, rather than what you lack, you can cultivate a sense of joy and appreciation that can lead to inspiration.

Another way to find inspiration in daily life is to seek out new experiences and perspectives. Try something new, like a new hobby or activity, or explore a new part of your city or town. By exposing yourself to new ideas and perspectives, you can broaden your horizons and find inspiration in unexpected places.

Finally, finding inspiration in daily life is about embracing your own unique perspective and voice. Don't be afraid to express yourself and share your ideas with the world. Your experiences and insights are valuable, and can inspire others in ways you may not even realize.

Remember, inspiration is not something that can be found outside of yourself - it comes from within. By being present, open, and grateful in your daily life, you can cultivate a sense of inspiration and motivation that can help you pursue your passions and achieve your dreams.

So I encourage you to embrace the journey towards finding inspiration in daily life. Take the time to appreciate the small things, seek out new experiences and perspectives, and embrace your own unique voice. You never know where inspiration may come from - it could be right in front of you, waiting to be discovered. Passion is a powerful force that can drive us towards our goals and dreams, and provide us with the motivation we need to overcome obstacles and challenges.

When we are truly passionate about something, it fuels us with a sense of purpose and direction. It gives us a reason to get out of bed in the morning, and to keep pushing forward even when things get tough.

Passion is not just a feeling, it is a force that can inspire us to take action towards our goals and dreams. It can help us to stay focused and motivated, even when we encounter setbacks or obstacles along the way.

So, never underestimate the power of passion in your life. Whether it is a passion for your work, your hobbies, or your relationships, allow it to fuel you with the motivation and energy you need to achieve greatness.

Remember, passion is not just a fleeting emotion - it is a force that can transform your life and give you the drive and determination you need to create a life of purpose and fulfillment. Passion is like a force of nature, a powerful energy that can propel us towards our greatest dreams and aspirations. It can inspire us to take action, to push ourselves beyond our limits, and to never give up on what we truly want.

When we are truly passionate about something, it fills us

with a sense of purpose and direction. It gives us a reason to keep going, even when the journey ahead seems long and difficult.

Passion can be a driving force in our lives, helping us to overcome obstacles and challenges with determination and resilience. It can light a fire within us, and push us to do more, be more, and achieve more than we ever thought possible.

So, if you have a passion burning inside you, don't ignore it or push it aside. Embrace it, nurture it, and let it guide you towards your greatest potential. Let it be the driving force that propels you towards your dreams, and the motivation that keeps you going when things get tough. Guiding yourself towards your passion can be a challenging journey, but it's also one of the most rewarding and fulfilling experiences you can have. It requires courage, determination, and a willingness to explore and discover what truly lights you up inside.

The first step in guiding yourself towards your passion is to take the time to reflect on your interests, values, and strengths. What do you enjoy doing? What are your core values and beliefs? What are you naturally good at? By exploring these questions, you can start to identify areas of your life that align with your passions.

Next, it's important to try new things and explore different opportunities. This can include taking classes, joining clubs or organizations, volunteering, or simply trying out new hobbies and activities. By stepping outside of your comfort zone and exploring new experiences, you may discover a passion that you never even knew existed.

It's also important to stay open-minded and curious. Don't be afraid to ask questions, to seek out new experiences, and to embrace the unknown. Remember, your passion may not reveal itself overnight - it may take time and patience to discover what truly lights you up inside.

And finally, don't be afraid to take action towards your passion. This may involve making bold decisions or taking risks, but it's important to trust your instincts and follow your heart. By taking action towards your passion, you can create a life that is aligned with your deepest values and aspirations, and experience a sense of purpose and fulfillment that is truly life-changing.

Remember, guiding yourself towards your passion is a journey - one that requires courage, patience, and a willingness to explore and discover. Finding courage can be a daunting task, but it's also one of the most rewarding and transformative experiences you can have. Courage is the fuel that drives us forward towards our dreams and aspirations, even in the face of fear and uncertainty.

The first step in finding courage is to acknowledge and accept your fears. We all experience fear at some point in our lives, and it's important to recognize that it's a natural part of the human experience. By accepting your fears, you can begin to understand them and work towards overcoming them.

Next, it's important to cultivate self-compassion and self-love. Remember that you are worthy and deserving of a life that is filled with joy, purpose, and meaning. By treating yourself with kindness and compassion, you can build the inner strength and resilience needed to face your fears and overcome obstacles.

It's also important to surround yourself with supportive and encouraging people. This can include friends, family members, mentors, or even support groups. By having a strong support network, you can draw strength and inspiration from those around you, and find the courage to pursue your dreams and aspirations.

And finally, it's important to take action towards your goals, even in the face of fear and uncertainty. This may involve taking risks or making bold decisions, but it's important to trust yourself and your instincts. Remember, the greatest growth and transformation often happens outside of our comfort zones. Controlling passion can be a tricky balance to achieve. On one hand, passion is what fuels us and drives us towards our goals and dreams. It's what makes us feel alive and gives us a sense of purpose and meaning. But on the other hand, too much passion can lead to burnout, overwhelm, and even negative consequences.

The key to controlling passion is to approach it with intention and balance. It's important to channel your passion in a way that aligns with your values and priorities, and to avoid letting it consume your life to the point where it becomes detrimental to your health and wellbeing.

One practical strategy for controlling passion is to set boundaries and prioritize self-care. This may mean taking breaks when you feel overwhelmed, delegating tasks to others, or setting limits on the amount of time and energy you devote to certain activities.

Another strategy is to cultivate mindfulness and self-awareness. By tuning into your thoughts, emotions, and physical sensations, you can gain a better understanding of when your passion is serving you and when it's becoming too much to handle. From there, you can make intentional choices about how to channel your passion in a healthy and sustainable way. Leaving our comfort zones can be scary and challenging, but it is often necessary for growth and personal development. It requires us to step into the unknown, to take risks, and to confront our fears and doubts. But when we do so, we open ourselves up to new opportunities, experiences, and perspectives that can enrich our lives in ways we never thought possible.

Remember, it's okay to feel uncomfortable or uncertain when leaving your comfort zone. It's a natural part of the process, and it's a sign that you are pushing yourself towards growth and new possibilities. Allow yourself to feel the discomfort, but don't let it hold you back from taking action towards your goals and dreams.

One practical strategy for leaving your comfort zone is to start small. Take small, intentional steps outside of your comfort zone, and gradually build up your confidence and comfort level. This can help to make the process feel more manageable and less overwhelming.

Another strategy is to cultivate a growth mindset. Embrace

challenges as opportunities for learning and growth, and view failure as a natural part of the process. By doing so, you can shift your perspective and approach to discomfort and uncertainty, and become more resilient and adaptable in the face of change. Finding freedom from ourselves can be a challenging but ultimately rewarding journey. It requires us to confront and challenge our own limiting beliefs and negative self-talk, and to cultivate a more compassionate and self-aware mindset. By learning to let go of self-judgment and embrace self-acceptance, we can free ourselves from the constraints of our own thoughts and behaviors, and live a more fulfilling and authentic life. Remember, the journey towards freedom from self is not easy, but with courage, perseverance, and self-compassion, it is possible. Embarking on the journey towards freedom from self can be a daunting task. It requires us to look deep within ourselves and confront the parts of us that we may not like or want to acknowledge. But it is also a journey that can bring immense growth and fulfillment. Imagine what it would feel like to be free from the weight of self-doubt and criticism, and to truly embrace and love ourselves for who we are. It may be a difficult road, but it is one that is worth taking. So have the courage to take that first step towards freedom, and know that you are capable of

overcoming any obstacle that may arise along the way

Chapter 10

THE INFLUENCE OF ENVIRONMENT

Have you ever felt weighed down by negativity, like you're surrounded by people and situations that drain your energy and dampen your spirits? It's a painful feeling, but the good news is that you have the power to surround yourself with positivity - and it all starts with your mindset.

Surrounding yourself with positivity is an emotional journey, one that requires a willingness to shift your perspective and seek out new opportunities and relationships. It's about focusing on the good in your life, and letting go of the things that hold you back.

One way to surround yourself with positivity is to practice gratitude. Take the time to appreciate the people and things in your life that bring you joy and fulfillment, and let go of the things that bring you down. By focusing on the positive, you can cultivate a sense of joy and optimism that can help you navigate even the toughest situations.

Another way to surround yourself with positivity is to seek out positive relationships and experiences.eeking out positive relationships can be a powerful way to cultivate a more positive mindset and improve your overall well-being. By surrounding yourself with people who uplift and support you, you can build a strong support network and experience greater joy and fulfillment in your life. Whether it's seeking out new friendships, deepening existing relationships, or seeking out professional networks and mentors, there are many ways to seek out positive relationships in your life. Remember, you deserve to be surrounded by people who bring out the best in you and support your growth and success. Don't be afraid to seek out those connections and invest in the relationships that bring you happiness and fulfillment. Surround yourself with people who uplift and inspire you, and seek out activities and environments that align with your values and aspirations. By surrounding yourself with positivity, you can create a sense of support and encouragement that can help you achieve your goals and overcome obstacles.

Finally, surrounding yourself with positivity is about

cultivating a positive mindset. Practice self-compassion and self-care, and focus on your strengths and accomplishments rather than your shortcomings and failures. By embracing a positive mindset, you can cultivate a sense of confidence and resilience that can help you overcome even the toughest challenges.

Remember, surrounding yourself with positivity is not about ignoring the challenges and difficulties in your life - it's about choosing to focus on the good, and letting that positivity guide your actions and mindset.

So I encourage you to embrace the journey towards surrounding yourself with positivity. Practice gratitude, seek out positive relationships and experiences, and cultivate a positive mindset. You have the power to create a life that is filled with joy, fulfillment, and positivity - all you have to do is start with your mindset.

Practicing Gratitude: Practicing gratitude is a powerful way to shift our mindset from one of scarcity and negativity to one of abundance and positivity. There are many simple but effective ways to incorporate gratitude into your daily life, such as keeping a gratitude journal, practicing mindfulness and being present in the moment, and expressing gratitude to others through acts of kindness and appreciation. By making gratitude a daily practice, we can cultivate a greater sense of joy, fulfillment, and contentment in our lives. Remember, gratitude is a practice, and like any practice, it takes time, effort, and consistency to see its benefits. So start small, be patient and compassionate with yourself, and watch as gratitude transforms your life in amazing ways.

Remember to be kind and gentle with yourself. Practicing self-compassion and self-care is essential to maintaining a positive mindset and overall well-being. Take time to prioritize your physical and emotional needs, and be patient and understanding with yourself during challenging times. Remember, you are deserving of love and care, and by practicing self-compassion and self-care, you can cultivate a more positive and fulfilling life. Self-love is a deep and profound sense of acceptance and appreciation for oneself. It means recognizing our own worth and value as individuals, and treating ourselves with kindness, compassion, and respect. Self-love involves embracing our strengths and imperfections, and learning to forgive ourselves for our mistakes and shortcomings. When we practice self-love, we create a foundation of confidence and self-assuredness that can help us navigate life's challenges with greater ease and grace. Remember, self-love is a journey, and it requires ongoing practice and self-reflection.

Positive affirmations:

1: I am worthy of love and respect.

You are truly worthy of love and respect, just as you are. You deserve to be treated with kindness and compassion, and to be surrounded by people who uplift and support you. Remember, your worthiness is not based on external factors or achievements, but simply on the fact that you are a unique and valuable human being. Believe in yourself, and know that you are deserving of all the love and respect in the world.

2:I choose to focus on the positive aspects of my life.

I am grateful for the many blessings in my life and I choose to focus on them. I know that by doing so, I am attracting more positivity and abundance into my life.

3: I am capable of achieving my goals and dreams.

Believe in yourself! You are capable of achieving greatness and making your dreams a reality. Trust in your abilities and know that with hard work and determination, anything is possible. Keep pushing forward and never give up on your aspirations.

4: I trust in my abilities and believe in myself.

Believing in myself gives me the confidence to pursue my dreams and overcome any obstacle. I trust in my abilities to navigate through challenges and to ultimately achieve success.

5: I am surrounded by love and support.

You are not alone, you are surrounded by the love and support of those around you. Believe in the power of community and lean on those who care about you. You are deserving of love and kindness.

6: I am grateful for all that I have in my life.

Expressing gratitude is a powerful tool for shifting your mindset to a more positive and fulfilling one. When you practice gratitude, you begin to notice and appreciate the blessings in your life, no matter how small they may seem. By affirming your gratitude regularly, you cultivate a sense of abundance and contentment, and you become more resilient in the face of challenges. Remember, even in difficult times, there is always something to be thankful for.

7: I choose to let go of negative thoughts and emotions.

I feel empowered as I release negative thoughts and

emotions, making room for positivity and growth in my life.

8: I am deserving of happiness and joy.

You are deserving of happiness and joy. You have the power to create a life that brings you fulfillment and contentment, and you are capable of achieving all that you desire. Trust in yourself and your abilities, and know that you are worthy of love, success, and abundance. Keep moving forward with positivity and optimism, and watch as your life transforms into one of beauty and meaning.

9: I embrace my unique qualities and strengths.

You are an amazing individual with unique qualities and strengths that make you special. Embrace those qualities and let them shine, for they are what make you who you are. Believe in yourself and your abilities, and never forget the value that you bring to the world.

10: I am open to new opportunities and experiences.

You are capable of embracing new opportunities and experiences. Your openness and willingness to try new things will lead to growth and new discoveries about yourself. Trust in your abilities and know that you are capable of achieving great things.

These are some positive affirmations, though yours may be different. Take the time to create your own personal affirmations that resonate with you and your goals. Whether it's reminding yourself of your worth, believing in your abilities, or focusing on gratitude and positivity, choose affirmations that uplift and motivate you. With regular practice, positive affirmations can help you cultivate a more positive and empowered mindset.

Chapter 11

OVERCOMING OBSTACLES

Have you ever found yourself procrastinating, putting off tasks that you know you should be doing? It's a frustrating feeling, but the good news is that you have the power to overcome procrastination - and it all starts with understanding the emotions that are driving it.

Procrastination is often driven by fear - fear of failure, fear of success, fear of the unknown. It's a natural human response to uncertainty and discomfort, but it can hold us back from achieving our goals and living our best lives.

Overcoming procrastination is an emotional journey, one that requires a willingness to face your fears and take action despite them. It's about recognizing the negative thought patterns that are driving your procrastination, and replacing them with positive self-talk and affirmations.

One way to overcome procrastination is to break tasks

down into smaller, more manageable steps. This can help to reduce feelings of overwhelm and make it easier to take action. Another way is to set deadlines and hold yourself accountable, either through a friend, mentor, or coach. This can help to create a sense of urgency and momentum that can push you towards action.

Finally, overcoming procrastination is about cultivating a sense of self-compassion and understanding. Be kind to yourself, and recognize that procrastination is a natural human response. Don't be too hard on yourself when you slip up, but instead, focus on the progress you've made and the steps you can take to move forward.

Remember, overcoming procrastination is not just about achieving external success - it's about cultivating a sense of empowerment and self-belief. When you take action despite your fears and doubts, you become stronger and more resilient.

So I encourage you to embrace the journey towards overcoming procrastination. Recognize the emotions that are driving your procrastination, and take action despite them. Break tasks down into smaller steps, set deadlines and hold yourself accountable, and cultivate a sense of self-compassion and understanding. You have the power to overcome procrastination and achieve your goals - all you have to do is take the first step.

Overcoming obstacles in life can be challenging, but it is possible with the right mindset and strategies. One important strategy is to approach obstacles with a growth mindset, seeing them as opportunities for growth and learning rather than insurmountable barriers.

Another helpful strategy is to break down the obstacle into smaller, more manageable steps, and to focus on taking one step at a time. This can help to prevent overwhelm and build momentum towards progress.

It can also be helpful to seek support and guidance from others, whether it's a trusted friend, family member, or professional. Having a supportive network can provide encouragement, motivation, and helpful insights for overcoming obstacles.

Finally, it's important to practice self-compassion and self-care during challenging times. This can involve engaging in self-care practices like meditation, exercise, or spending time in nature, as well as cultivating a compassionate and understanding mindset towards yourself. Nature has a unique ability to ground and center us, allowing us to connect with the present moment and find inner peace. Whether it's taking a walk in the park, going for a hike in the mountains, or simply sitting in a quiet place surrounded by nature, spending time in nature can be a powerful tool for overcoming obstacles in life. The natural beauty and rhythms of nature can help us to find perspective and clarity, and to let go of the stresses and worries of daily life. So if you're feeling overwhelmed or stuck, consider taking a break and spending some time in nature - you may be surprised at the positive impact it can have on your mindset and well-being.

Negative Self-talk:

Negative self-talk can be damaging to our mental health and well-being, but it can also be used as a tool for grounding and self-awareness. When we become aware of our negative self-talk patterns, we can begin to challenge and reframe them, and use them as a cue to ground ourselves in the present moment. By acknowledging our thoughts and feelings without judgment, we can begin to cultivate a sense of self-compassion and self-awareness, which can help us to navigate life's challenges with greater resilience and positivity. Remember, using negative self-talk in a healthy way requires a commitment to self-awareness and self-compassion, and may require support from others, such as a therapist or trusted friend.

Dealing with Negative Self-Image:

Dealing with negative self-image can be a challenging journey, but it is possible with the right mindset and strategies. One way to start is by practicing self-compassion and reframing negative self-talk. Instead of focusing on your flaws and shortcomings, focus on your strengths and accomplishments, and speak to yourself with kindness and encouragement.

Another helpful strategy is to surround yourself with positive and supportive people, who will uplift and motivate you towards positivity. It is also important to engage in activities that bring you joy and fulfillment, whether it be a hobby or spending time in nature.

Remember that building a positive self-image takes time and effort, but by committing to the journey and being kind to yourself, you can learn to embrace your unique qualities

Gaining Willpower to follow through:

Gaining willpower can be a challenging process, but it's an essential component of achieving our goals and living a fulfilling life. One of the key strategies for building willpower is to start small and gradually increase the difficulty of our challenges. This can help us to build momentum and confidence, and to gradually strengthen our willpower over time.

Another strategy is to stay focused on our goals and to remind ourselves of why we started in the first place. By staying connected to our deepest values and motivations, we can tap into a powerful source of inspiration and drive that can help us to overcome even the toughest challenges.

Additionally, practicing self-care and self-compassion can be helpful in building willpower. By taking care of our physical and emotional needs, we can create a foundation of strength and resilience that can help us to stay focused and motivated in the face of obstacles. as you continue to grow it is beneficial to be It's important to be aware of narcissistic thoughts and behaviors, as they can be harmful to both ourselves and those around us. When we constantly focus on our own needs and desires, we may become insensitive to the needs and feelings of others, which can damage our relationships and lead to feelings of loneliness and isolation. By cultivating a more empathetic and compassionate mindset, we can overcome narcissistic tendencies and build stronger, more fulfilling connections with the people in our lives.

Remember, true happiness and fulfillment come not from our own achievements and successes, but from the positive impact we have on others. Meeting your needs unselfishly is about finding a balance between taking care of yourself and considering the needs of others. It means prioritizing self-care and self-compassion, while also being mindful of how your actions and decisions impact those around you. By approaching your own needs with kindness and understanding, and by seeking out opportunities to help and support others, you can create a more fulfilling and meaningful life for yourself and those around you. Remember, meeting your needs unselfishly is not just about doing what feels good in the moment, but about making intentional choices that benefit both yourself and the greater good. in the end life is all about Life is full of obstacles, and we all face them in different forms and at different times. Some of these obstacles can seem insurmountable, and we may feel like giving up. But it is during these times of challenge that we have the opportunity to grow and to become stronger.

When I was a child, I faced a significant obstacle that could have defined the rest of my life. I was born with a hearing impairment, and my parents were told that I would never be able to speak or hear properly. My mother, however, refused to accept this prognosis and spent countless hours working with me to teach me how to speak and communicate. It was a long and difficult journey, but I eventually overcame this obstacle and was able to live a normal life.

As I grew older, I faced many other obstacles, both personal and professional. I lost loved ones, experienced heartbreak, and struggled to find my place in the world. But through it all, I learned that overcoming obstacles is essential for personal growth and success.

One of the most significant obstacles I faced was when I decided to start my own business. I had no experience, no contacts, and no idea where to begin. I faced countless rejections and setbacks, but I refused to give up. I worked tirelessly to learn everything I could about entrepreneurship and slowly built my business from the ground up.

Through this experience, I learned that the key to overcoming obstacles is to stay focused on your goals and to never give up. It's easy to become discouraged when things don't go as planned, but it's essential to keep pushing forward, even when the road ahead seems uncertain.

Overcoming obstacles also requires a willingness to learn and to adapt. When we face challenges, we have the opportunity to learn new skills and to develop new ways of thinking. It's important to embrace these opportunities and to use them to our advantage.

In the end, the most important lesson I learned is that overcoming obstacles is not about achieving perfection or avoiding failure. It's about developing resilience and the strength to keep going, even when the odds are against us. It's about recognizing that obstacles are a natural part of life and that we have the power to overcome them.

As we navigate through life's challenges, it's important to remember that we are not alone. We all face obstacles, and we all have the power to overcome them. By staying focused on our goals, embracing new opportunities, and never giving up, we can achieve great things and live a life of purpose and fulfillment.

Chapter 12

THE POWER OF GRATITUDE

Have you ever faced a challenge or setback that left you feeling defeated and discouraged? It's a painful feeling, but the good news is that you have the power to build resilience - and it all starts with your mindset.

Resilience is the ability to bounce back from adversity, to overcome obstacles and setbacks with grace and determination. It's a quality that can help you navigate even the toughest situations, and emerge stronger and more resilient on the other side.

Building resilience is an emotional journey, one that requires a willingness to face your fears and doubts, and to embrace the challenges and opportunities that come your way. It's about cultivating a sense of inner strength and confidence that can help you navigate even the toughest situations.

One way to build resilience is to cultivate a growth mindset.

Embrace the idea that your abilities and talents can be developed through hard work, dedication, and perseverance. Focus on the things you can control, and let go of the things you can't. By embracing a growth mindset, you can cultivate a sense of confidence and resilience that can help you overcome even the toughest challenges.

Another way to build resilience is to practice self-care and self-compassion. Take care of yourself physically, mentally, and emotionally, and give yourself the time and space you need to rest and recharge. Be kind to yourself, and recognize that setbacks and failures are a natural part of the human experience.

Finally, building resilience is about seeking out support and guidance when you need it. Surround yourself with positive relationships and experiences, and seek out mentors or coaches who can help guide you through tough times. By building a sense of support and encouragement around you, you can cultivate a sense of resilience and inner strength that can help you navigate even the toughest situations.

Remember, building resilience is not just about achieving external success - it's about cultivating a sense of inner strength and confidence that can help you navigate all areas of your life.

When you approach challenges with a resilient mindset, you become more confident, more resilient, and more fulfilled.

So I encourage you to embrace the journey towards building resilience. Cultivate a growth mindset, practice self-care and self-compassion, and seek out support and guidance when you need it. You have the power to build resilience and overcome even the toughest challenges. Gratitude is a powerful emotion that has the ability to transform our lives in countless ways. It is the feeling of appreciation and thankfulness for the people, experiences, and things that bring joy and meaning to our lives.

Growing up, I always took the blessings in my life for granted. I was privileged and had everything I needed, but I failed to recognize and appreciate the love and support of my family and friends. It wasn't until I experienced a difficult time in my life that I realized the importance of gratitude.

I had just gone through a painful breakup and was struggling with feelings of sadness and loneliness. But then I started to focus on the things that I was grateful for, such as my health, my family, and my career. As I shifted my focus from what was missing in my life to what I had, I felt a sense of peace and contentment that I had never experienced before.

Through this experience, I learned that gratitude has the power to change our perspective and to bring us joy and fulfillment. When we focus on what we are thankful for, we open ourselves up to the abundance and blessings that surround us.

Gratitude also has the ability to improve our relationships with others. When we express gratitude for the people in our lives, we deepen our connection and strengthen our bonds. It allows us to recognize the efforts and sacrifices of others and to appreciate the impact they have on our lives.

Furthermore, gratitude has been shown to have numerous physical and mental health benefits. Studies have found that those who regularly practice gratitude have lower levels of stress, improved sleep quality, and increased feelings of happiness and well-being.

In a world that often emphasizes what we don't have, it can be easy to forget the abundance that surrounds us. But by cultivating a practice of gratitude, we can transform our lives and our relationships in meaningful ways.

As I continue to practice gratitude in my daily life, I am constantly reminded of the power it holds. It has allowed me to find joy in the simplest moments and to appreciate the people in my life in new and profound ways. I am grateful for the transformative power of gratitude and the impact it has had on my life.

It's easy to get caught up in the hustle and bustle of daily life and to overlook the abundance that surrounds us. We are bombarded with messages that tell us we need more, we need to be better, and we need to do more. In the midst of all this noise, it's easy to forget the beauty and blessings that we already have in our lives.

It wasn't until I went through a difficult time in my life that I discovered the transformative power of gratitude. I had just lost my job and was struggling to make ends meet. I felt overwhelmed and anxious about the future. But then I started to focus on the things that I was grateful for, like my health, my family, and my friends.

As I shifted my focus from what I didn't have to what I did have, I felt a sense of peace and contentment wash over me. I realized that even in the midst of difficult circumstances, there is always something to be thankful for. By cultivating a practice of gratitude, I was able to transform my perspective and to find joy in the simplest moments.

Gratitude has the power to transform our relationships as well. When we express gratitude for the people in our lives, we deepen our connection and strengthen our bonds. It allows us to recognize the efforts and sacrifices of others and to appreciate the impact they have on our lives. In a world that often values individualism and competition, gratitude reminds us of our interconnectedness and our shared humanity.

Moreover, cultivating a practice of gratitude has been shown to have numerous physical and mental health benefits. Studies have found that those who regularly practice gratitude have lower levels of stress, improved sleep quality, and increased feelings of happiness and well-being.

In a society that often emphasizes what we don't have, it can be easy to forget the abundance that surrounds us. But by cultivating a practice of gratitude, we can transform our lives and our relationships in meaningful ways. It allows us to see the beauty and blessings in our lives and to appreciate the people who make our lives worth living.

As I continue to practice gratitude in my daily life, I am constantly reminded of its transformative power. I am grateful for the beauty and abundance that surrounds me, and for the people who make my life rich and fulfilling.

Chapter 13

SUSTAINING MOTIVATION FOR THE LONG HAUL

Have you ever found yourself struggling with motivation, feeling stuck in a rut and unable to find the drive to pursue your passions? It's a difficult feeling, but the good news is that mindfulness can play a powerful role in cultivating motivation and helping you find the inspiration you need to move forward.

Mindfulness is the practice of being present in the moment, fully engaged with your thoughts, feelings, and surroundings. It's a powerful tool that can help you cultivate a sense of clarity and focus, and can be a key factor in building motivation and resilience.

One way that mindfulness can help with motivation is by helping you connect with your innermost desires and values. By taking the time to reflect on what truly matters to you, you can gain a deeper understanding of your goals and aspirations, and find the inspiration you need to pursue them with passion and determination.

Another way that mindfulness can help with motivation is by helping you cultivate a sense of calm and centeredness. By practicing mindfulness, you can learn to manage stress and anxiety more effectively, and find the inner strength and resilience you need to overcome obstacles and setbacks.

Finally, mindfulness can help with motivation by helping you stay present and engaged in the moment. When you are fully engaged with your thoughts, feelings, and surroundings, you are more likely to find inspiration and motivation in the world around you, and to pursue your passions with a sense of purpose and determination.

Remember, mindfulness is not a magic solution for all of life's challenges - it's a powerful tool that can help you cultivate motivation and resilience in the face of adversity. By practicing mindfulness on a regular basis, you can cultivate a sense of clarity and focus, and find the inspiration you need to pursue your passions and achieve your goals.

So I encourage you to embrace the role of mindfulness in motivation. Take the time to reflect on your goals and values, cultivate a sense of calm and centeredness, and stay present and engaged in the moment. You have the power to cultivate motivation and resilience through the practice of mindfulness - all you have to do is take the first step. I am so excited to share with you the incredible potential of mindfulness in cultivating motivation and resilience. The journey towards your goals can be challenging, but by embracing mindfulness, you can tap into a sense of inner strength and purpose that will propel you forward.

It's not always easy to stay motivated, especially when faced with obstacles or setbacks. But when you take the time to reflect on your goals and values, and cultivate a sense of calm and centeredness through mindfulness, you will find that you have the power to overcome any challenge.

I know that sometimes it can be hard to make the first step towards a new practice or habit, but trust me when I say that the rewards are immeasurable. By embracing mindfulness, you will not only become more motivated and resilient, but you will also experience greater peace, joy, and fulfillment in your daily life.

Again I encourage you to take that first step today. Set aside a few minutes to practice mindfulness, whether it's through meditation, mindful breathing, or simply being present in the moment. With each moment of mindfulness, you will be cultivating the inner resources you need to achieve your goals and overcome any obstacle.

You have the power within you to create the life you desire. So let's take this journey towards mindful motivation and resilience together, one step at a time. Have you ever heard the saying that you are the sum total of the five people you spend time with? It's a powerful reminder of the impact that the people around us can have on our lives.

The truth is, the people we surround ourselves with can either lift us up or drag us down. They can inspire us to be our best selves, or they can hold us back from reaching our full potential.

That's why it's so important to be intentional about the people we allow into our lives. We should seek out those who share our values, support our goals, and encourage us to grow and evolve.

It's not always easy to let go of relationships that no longer serve us, but sometimes it's necessary for our own growth and well-being. We owe it to ourselves to surround ourselves with people who lift us up and help us become the best version of ourselves.

So, take a moment to reflect on the people in your life. Are they helping you grow and evolve, or are they holding you back? If you find that you're spending time with people who are not aligned with your values and goals, it may be time to make some changes.

Remember, you deserve to surround yourself with people who support and uplift you. You have the power to choose the people you spend time with, so choose wisely. Let's surround ourselves with positive influences that will help us reach our full potential.

Setting Boundaries:

Setting and maintaining healthy boundaries is an essential part of self-care and self-respect. It's about knowing our limits and communicating them to others in a clear and compassionate way.

We all have different needs and preferences, and it's important to honor those needs and preferences in our relationships with others. When we set boundaries, we are sending a message to the world that we value ourselves and our well-being.

However, setting boundaries can be challenging, especially if we're used to putting other people's needs ahead of our own. It can feel uncomfortable to say "no" or to assert ourselves in a situation where we feel vulnerable or uncertain.

But remember, setting boundaries is not about being selfish or uncaring. It's about taking care of ourselves so that we can show up fully for others in a healthy and sustainable way. When we respect our own boundaries, we teach others to respect them as well, which can lead to deeper and more fulfilling relationships.

Of course, maintaining boundaries can be an ongoing process, and it's important to be flexible and open to feedback from others. Sometimes we may need to adjust our boundaries to better serve our needs, or to accommodate the needs of others in a respectful and healthy way.

So, I encourage you to take some time to reflect on your own needs and boundaries, and to communicate them to others in a clear and compassionate way. Remember, you deserve to be treated with respect and kindness, and it's up to you to create the relationships and environments that support your well-being.

Chapter 14

ACHIEVING SUCCESS

Have you ever achieved a goal or milestone, only to feel like you didn't deserve to celebrate it? It's a common feeling, but the truth is that celebrating your successes is an important part of the journey towards achieving your goals - and it can be a powerful source of motivation and inspiration.

Celebrating your successes is an emotional journey, one that requires a willingness to acknowledge your accomplishments and to give yourself credit for the hard work and dedication you've put in. It's about recognizing that every step forward, no matter how small, is a step in the right direction.

One way to celebrate your successes is to take the time to reflect on your journey so far. Think about the challenges you've faced and the obstacles you've overcome, and give yourself credit for the progress you've made. By reflecting on your journey, you can cultivate a sense of gratitude and appreciation for the hard work and dedication that has brought you to this point.

Another way to celebrate your successes is to share them with others. Surround yourself with positive relationships and experiences, and share your accomplishments with friends, family, or mentors who can provide support and encouragement. By sharing your successes with others, you can cultivate a sense of pride and confidence in your abilities, and inspire others to pursue their own goals and dreams.

Finally, celebrating your successes is about practicing self-compassion and self-care. Take the time to acknowledge your accomplishments, and give yourself permission to celebrate them. Treat yourself to something special, whether it's a nice meal, a relaxing day at the spa, or a simple moment of quiet reflection. By practicing self-care and self-compassion, you can cultivate a sense of inner strength and resilience that can help you achieve even greater success in the future.

Remember, celebrating your successes is not about arrogance or selfishness - it's about acknowledging the hard work and dedication that has brought you to this point, and giving yourself the credit you deserve. When you celebrate your successes, you become more motivated, more confident, and more fulfilled - all of which can help you achieve even greater success in the future.

So I encourage you to embrace the journey towards celebrating your successes. Reflect on your journey, share your accomplishments with others, and practice self-compassion and self-care. You have the power to cultivate a sense of pride and confidence in your abilities, and to achieve even greater success in the future. All you have to do is take the first step.

Have you ever felt like you were on your own, trying to achieve your goals and dreams without any support or guidance? It's a difficult feeling, but the truth is that seeking support and accountability can be a powerful tool in helping you achieve your goals and stay motivated along the way.

Seeking support and accountability is an emotional journey, one that requires a willingness to be vulnerable and to ask for help when you need it. It's about recognizing that we all need support and guidance from time to time, and that it's okay to ask for help.

One way to seek support and accountability is to surround yourself with positive relationships and experiences. Find people who uplift and inspire you, and seek out mentors or coaches who can provide guidance and support as you pursue your goals. By surrounding yourself with positivity, you can cultivate a sense of encouragement and motivation that can help you stay on track and achieve your goals.

Another way to seek support and accountability is to set up systems of accountability for yourself. Find someone you trust and respect, and ask them to hold you accountable for your progress towards your goals. Whether it's a weekly check-in, a progress report, or a simple conversation about your progress, having someone to hold you accountable can be a powerful motivator in helping you stay focused and on track.

Finally, seeking support and accountability is about practicing self-compassion and self-care. Recognize that setbacks and failures are a natural part of the journey towards achieving your goals, and be kind to yourself as you navigate these challenges. By practicing self-compassion and self-care, you can cultivate a sense of inner strength and resilience that can help you overcome even the toughest obstacles.

Remember, seeking support and accountability is not a sign of weakness - it's a sign of strength and determination. When you surround yourself with positive relationships and experiences, set up systems of accountability, and practice self-compassion and self-care, you can achieve even greater success and fulfillment in your life.

So I encourage you to embrace the journey towards seeking support and accountability. Surround yourself with positivity, set up systems of accountability, and practice self-compassion and self-care. You have the power to achieve your goals and dreams - all you have to do is ask for the support and guidance you need along the way.

Success means different things to different people, but regardless of how we define it, we all have the capacity to achieve it. Here are some different ways that you can pursue success in your own life:

Set clear goals: Success starts with a clear vision of what you want to achieve. Set specific, measurable goals that align with your values and aspirations.

Take action: Once you've set your goals, it's time to take action. Break down your goals into smaller, achievable steps, and take consistent action towards them.

Embrace failure: Failure is an inevitable part of the journey towards success. Instead of letting failure hold you back, use it as an opportunity to learn, grow, and pivot towards a new direction.

Cultivate resilience: Success requires resilience - the ability to bounce back from setbacks and keep moving forward. Cultivate resilience by practicing self-care, surrounding yourself with supportive people, and developing a growth mindset.

Keep learning: Success is an ongoing process of learning and growth. Seek out opportunities to expand your knowledge and skills, whether it's through formal education, mentorship, or self-study.

Take calculated risks: Success often requires taking risks and stepping outside of your comfort zone. Make informed decisions and take calculated risks that align with your goals and values.

Network and build relationships: Success is often a collaborative effort, and building strong relationships can open doors and create opportunities. Network with others in your field, and be open to building new connections.

Be persistent: Success is rarely achieved overnight. It takes persistence and determination to overcome obstacles and achieve your goals. Stay focused, stay motivated, and never give up.

Remember, success is not just about achieving external

markers of achievement, but also about feeling fulfilled, happy, and aligned with your values and purpose. So, find what success means to you and pursue it with passion, determination, and joy. Success and motivation go hand in hand. When we are motivated, we are driven to take action towards our goals, and this momentum can help us achieve success in our lives.

But what is motivation, and how do we cultivate it? Motivation is the inner drive that propels us towards our goals, and it can come from a variety of sources - from our personal values and passions to external rewards and recognition.

To cultivate motivation, it's important to first get clear on what we want to achieve. Set specific, measurable goals that align with your values and aspirations, and break them down into smaller, achievable steps.

Next, focus on the why behind your goals. What is motivating you to pursue these goals, and how will achieving them impact your life and the lives of those around you? Connect with the emotional and psychological rewards of achieving your goals, and use this as fuel to keep going.

Remember, motivation is not a constant state - it ebbs and flows over time. When you experience setbacks or obstacles, it's important to tap into your resilience and keep moving forward. Celebrate small wins along the way, and use them as inspiration to keep going.

Ultimately, success is not just about achieving external markers of achievement, but also about feeling fulfilled, happy, and aligned with your values and purpose. When we cultivate motivation from within, we can tap into our full potential and create a life that is truly meaningful and fulfilling.

So, I encourage you to take the first step towards cultivating motivation and achieving success in your own life. Connect with your passions, set clear goals, and take consistent action towards them. Remember, you have the power within you to create a life that is full of joy, purpose, and success.

Chapter 15

MOTIVATIONAL LIFESTYLE

Have you ever felt like motivation was something that came and went, rather than a consistent part of your life? It's a common feeling, but the good news is that you have the power to make motivation a lifestyle - something that is woven into the fabric of your daily life and routine.

Making motivation a lifestyle is an emotional journey, one that requires a commitment to cultivating positive habits and behaviors that support your goals and aspirations. It's about recognizing that motivation is not just a feeling - it's a way of being and living in the world.

One way to make motivation a lifestyle is to focus on building habits that support your goals and aspirations. Whether it's exercising regularly, eating healthy, or dedicating time each day to pursuing your passions, building positive habits and routines can help you stay motivated and on track towards your goals.

Another way to make motivation a lifestyle is to cultivate a growth mindset. Embrace challenges and setbacks as opportunities for growth and learning, and see the possibilities and opportunities that lie ahead. By cultivating a growth mindset, you can approach life with a sense of curiosity and wonder, and find the motivation and inspiration you need to pursue your dreams.

Finally, making motivation a lifestyle is about practicing self-care and self-compassion. Take care of yourself physically, mentally, and emotionally, and give yourself the time and space you need to rest and recharge. Be kind to yourself, and recognize that setbacks and failures are a natural part of the human experience.

Remember, making motivation a lifestyle is not just about achieving external success - it's about cultivating a sense of inner strength and resilience that can help you navigate all areas of your life. When you make motivation a lifestyle, you become more confident, more resilient, and more fulfilled.

So I encourage you to embrace the journey towards making motivation a lifestyle. Build positive habits, cultivate a growth mindset, and practice self-care and self-compassion. You have the power to make motivation a consistent part of your life - all you have to do is take the first step.

Living a motivational lifestyle is about cultivating a sense of purpose, passion, and joy in all aspects of your life. It's about waking up each day with a sense of excitement and energy, and approaching each moment with intention and enthusiasm.

But how do we create a motivational lifestyle? Here are some key steps:

Define your values and passions: What drives you? What brings you joy? Connect with your innermost values and passions, and use them as a guidepost for your daily choices and actions.

1: Set clear goals: Identify specific, measurable goals that align with your values and passions, and break them down into smaller, achievable steps.

Surround yourself with positivity: Seek out relationships and environments that uplift and inspire you. Surround yourself with positive influences that encourage growth and possibility.

Embrace challenges and failures: Living a motivational lifestyle means embracing challenges and setbacks as opportunities for growth and learning. Use failures as a chance to learn and pivot towards a new direction. Dear reader,

Embracing challenges and failures is an essential part of living a motivational lifestyle. It can be difficult to face setbacks and obstacles, but when we approach them with a growth mindset, we open ourselves up to new opportunities for learning and growth.

Instead of letting failures hold us back, we can use them as a chance to learn and pivot towards a new direction. We can ask ourselves what went wrong, what we can do differently in the future, and how we can use this experience to become stronger and more resilient.

Of course, embracing challenges and failures is easier said than done. It can be hard to let go of our attachment to a certain outcome, or to face the disappointment and frustration that comes with setbacks.

But remember, living a motivational lifestyle is not about achieving perfection or success without any obstacles. It's about finding purpose and joy in the journey, and using each experience - whether it's a success or a failure - as an opportunity for growth and learning.

So, I encourage you to embrace challenges and failures as

part of your journey towards a motivational lifestyle. Approach them with curiosity and an open mind, and use them as a chance to learn and pivot towards a new direction. With each setback, you'll be building resilience, wisdom, and strength that will propel you towards even greater success and fulfillment.

Remember, you have the power within you to overcome any challenge and achieve any goal. Let's embrace the challenges and failures of life with grace, resilience, and determination.

2: Practice self-care: Prioritize your own physical, emotional, and mental well-being. Take time to care for yourself through exercise, healthy eating, rest, and relaxation. Practicing self-care is an essential part of living a motivational lifestyle. It's about prioritizing your own physical, emotional, and mental well-being, so that you can show up fully for yourself and for others.

Taking care of yourself may sound simple, but it can be difficult to prioritize amidst the demands of everyday life. However, when we make self-care a priority, we create a foundation of strength and resilience that helps us navigate life's challenges with grace and ease.

Self-care can take many different forms, from exercise and healthy eating to rest and relaxation. It's about finding the activities and practices that nourish your mind, body, and soul, and making them a regular part of your routine.

When we practice self-care, we are sending a powerful message to ourselves and to the world that we value our own well-being. We are saying that we are worthy of love, care, and attention, and that we are committed to showing up as our best selves.

So, I encourage you to prioritize self-care in your own life. Take time to exercise, eat healthy, rest, and engage in activities that bring you joy and fulfillment. Remember, self-care is not selfish - it's an essential part of living a happy, healthy, and fulfilling life.

With each act of self-care, you are creating a foundation of strength, resilience, and motivation that will help you achieve your goals and live a life of purpose and passion. So, let's make self-care a priority and show ourselves the love and care we deserve.

3: Stay open to new experiences: Living a motivational lifestyle means staying curious and open to new experiences. Be willing to step outside of your comfort zone and try new things. Staying open to new experiences is a key part of living a motivational lifestyle. It's about staying curious, adventurous, and open to the possibilities that life has to offer.

When we stay open to new experiences, we are embracing the unknown and stepping outside of our comfort zones. We are saying yes to opportunities that may challenge us, but also have the potential to bring us joy, growth, and fulfillment.

Of course, staying open to new experiences can be scary. It means facing the unknown and letting go of our attachment to what is familiar and safe. But when we approach life with a sense of curiosity and adventure, we open ourselves up to new perspectives, new ideas, and new ways of being.

So, I encourage you to stay open to new experiences in your own life. Be willing to try new things, meet new people, and explore new places. Take risks, challenge yourself, and embrace the unexpected.

Remember, living a motivational lifestyle is not about playing it safe or sticking to what is comfortable. It's about finding joy, purpose, and growth in all aspects of your life. By staying open to new experiences, you are expanding your horizons and creating a life that is full of adventure, possibility, and motivation.

With each new experience, you are opening yourself up to the infinite possibilities that life has to offer. So, let's embrace the unknown, step outside of our comfort zones, and live a life that is full of curiosity, adventure, and motivation.

4: Remember, living a motivational lifestyle is not about achieving perfection or success on someone else's terms. It's about creating a life that is aligned with your own values and passions, and finding joy and fulfillment in the journey. It's easy to get caught up in the pursuit of external markers of success - a high-paying job, a perfect relationship, a beautiful home. But living a motivational lifestyle is not about achieving perfection or success on someone else's terms.

Instead, it's about creating a life that is aligned with your own values and passions, and finding joy and fulfillment in the journey. It's about defining success on your own terms, and pursuing goals that are meaningful and fulfilling to you.

When we focus on creating a life that aligns with our own values and passions, we tap into a sense of purpose and fulfillment that cannot be achieved through external markers of success. We create a life that is rich with meaning, joy, and motivation, and we inspire others to do the same.

So, I encourage you to take the time to define what success means to you. What are your core values and passions? What brings you joy and fulfillment? Once you have a clear sense of what matters most to you, you can begin to pursue goals and activities that align with those values and passions.

Remember, living a motivational lifestyle is not about achieving someone else's idea of success. It's about creating a life that is true to who you are, and finding joy and fulfillment in the journey. So, let's define success on our own terms, and create lives that are full of purpose, passion, and motivation.

So, I encourage you to take the first step towards living a motivational lifestyle. Connect with your innermost values and passions, and set clear goals that align with them. Surround yourself with positivity, embrace challenges and failures as opportunities for growth, and prioritize your own well-being. With each step, you'll be creating a life that is full of purpose, joy, and motivation.

EL FIN

MOTIVATION: FINDING SUCCESS

Dear Reader: Thank you for joining me on this journey. With great care and Love I hope that this book, as short as it is, helps you to achieve all of your dreams.

Sincerely: A.S.